INFLAMMATION ERASED:

Naturally Fight & Reverse Damaging Inflammatory Effects in Your Body

Susan Patterson
(B.A., CBHC, CMTA)

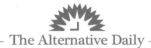

The Alternative Daily

Table of Contents

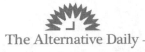

INFLAMMATION ERASED:

NATURALLY FIGHT & REVERSE DAMAGING INFLAMMATORY EFFECTS IN YOUR BODY

Introduction

*A*cute inflammation, also known as "healthy inflammation," is a self-defense mechanism initiated by the body as a means of protection. The purpose of this type of inflammation is to remove harmful stimuli such as damaged cells, pathogens, and irritants, so that the body can begin the healing process.

Chronic inflammation, also known as "unhealthy inflammation," on the other hand, can cause widespread damage and trigger a host of dangerous conditions. If you suffer from chronic inflammation, the time to act is now—before things get out of hand.

This book contains a wealth of knowledge about chronic inflammation. Our goal is to provide you with the facts so that you can make informed decisions about your health.

Our team of dedicated researchers, writers and editors have compiled the most up-to-date information within this book, because we truly believe that moving towards a place of optimal health and well-being is a journey well worth taking.

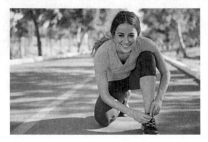

Let us help you along the way,

The Alternative Daily Team

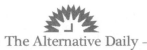

Chapter One
Facts and Figures

Interesting facts about inflammation

Did you know?

- The groundwork for a lot of the key research behind the current medical understanding of inflammation was performed by Elie Metchnikoff and Paul Ehrlich, who shared a Nobel Prize for Medicine for their work in 1908.

- While inflammation is an innately protective response by the immune system, if the reaction persists and becomes chronic, it can be highly damaging to the body.

- Many people experience chronic, low-grade inflammation for many years before it is identified as the problem—making this an especially dangerous threat to health.

- Low-level, chronic inflammation is sometimes referred to as "para-inflammation."

- Chronic inflammation is often mistaken as normal aging—when really, the aging process may not be quite as severe or damaging if inflammation were mitigated.

- Inflammation can occur anywhere in the body—from the skin down through to the deepest internal organs and tissues of the body. In some cases, it occurs throughout many of the body's systems.

- According to a body of research, including studies performed by the Centers for Disease Control and Prevention, low-level inflammation is a factor in seven of the ten leading causes of death in the United States.

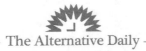

- Inflammation can be greatly worsened by stress. When levels of cortisol, aka the "stress hormone" are high, inflammation thrives.

- Some markers of inflammation, including C-reactive protein and interleukins, can be detected by blood tests. However, some of these tests may be expensive, and many people do not think to have them done until symptoms of autoimmune illness are already present.

- Many health professionals do not readily test for chronic inflammation unless requested to do so, or until certain symptoms are present—yet another reason why inflammation can go on for many years before it is noticed.

- Non-steroidal anti-inflammatory drugs (NSAIDs) are commonly prescribed or recommended to treat inflammation; however, these drugs can have many side effects, especially on the digestive system, and therefore a natural solution may be safer, and is often more effective.

- Age is a factor in chronic inflammation, so older individuals may be more susceptible to its worsening effects.

- Obesity is also a factor in chronic inflammation. Therefore, getting to a healthy weight—safely and through proper nutrition and exercise—may reduce the risk of chronic inflammation significantly.

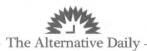

- Researchers are exploring the connection between inflammatory gum disease and heart disease. Some hypothesize that bacteria in the gums may travel to the heart through the bloodstream and contribute to cardiovascular problems.

- Consuming a diet rich in antioxidants can help to curb chronic inflammation, thereby potentially protecting your entire body from harm.

- Not getting enough sleep—seven to eight hours is the generally accepted guideline—may also contribute to inflammation, so there is significant harm in missing out on those necessary hours of shut-eye.

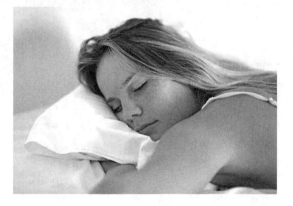

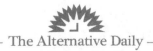

Chapter Two
The Good and the Bad

While they are both reactions by the immune system characterized by warmth and swelling, there is a world of difference between acute and chronic inflammation. The former protects our health, while the latter contributes to destroying it.

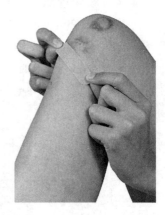

The good: acute inflammation is a natural defense against invasion

We've all had cuts, scrapes, and other injuries during the course of our lives—and it's easy to see the body's immediate response to this kind of damage. The area becomes red, swollen, painful and warm to the touch. If the injury is on a joint or muscle, that joint or muscle may become stiff and not move very easily. This is acute inflammation.

Acute inflammation occurs when the white blood cells of the body rush to the scene of an injury, or an invasion by a foreign substance (i.e., bacteria, virus, heavy metal), in an effort to protect us. Upon sensing the threat, the white blood cells release certain chemicals, which perform several protective functions.

Firstly, they aid the body in removing the invader, along with damaged or dead tissues. They also help to prevent the damage from spreading to other tissues, and help the body to repair the damage that has been done. Because of these functions, acute inflammation is a highly important function of the body—it keeps us safe from the damage of injury, as well as from pathogens which may harm us.

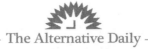

Along with redness, swelling, stiffness, and impaired motion in the injured area, acute inflammation can cause pain—both in the area and in surrounding nerves. The injured area may also become warm as a result of increased blood flow (those white blood cells have to arrive somehow). In the case of an invading pathogen, acute inflammation can feel quite similar to the flu—sometimes causing fever, headache, chills and fatigue. Loss of appetite can also occur.

While all of these symptoms of acute inflammation can surely be uncomfortable, it's actually your body doing you a favor. Without the acute inflammatory response of the immune system, we would suffer great harm from injuries and pathogens. It may not be fun, but it's a positive immunological response.

The main noteworthy characteristic of acute inflammation, besides its protective functions, is that once the injury is healed, or the pathogen in question has been destroyed, it subsides, and the body's function returns to normal.

The bad: chronic inflammation occurs when systems go awry

While acute inflammation serves to protect the body and its cells, chronic inflammation does quite the opposite, and can lead to severe system-wide damage over time.

Chronic inflammation occurs when the body's cells are stressed—by internal or external factors. It can also occur when white blood cells perceive a foreign invader that isn't there. An inflammatory response is triggered, sometimes in one area of the body and sometimes throughout the entire body. However, unlike acute inflammation, it does not dissipate, but rather lingers, wreaking havoc.

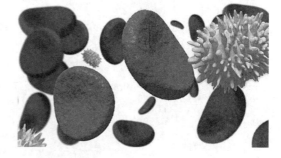

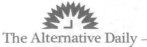

This type of inflammation can go unnoticed for a long time, as it may cause generalized discomfort that is not easily associated with inflammation. In some cases, symptoms of chronic inflammation may be dismissed as normal signs of the aging process, and are therefore overlooked until the inflammation has already caused significant harm.

This is known as "low-grade" chronic inflammation, and it may become severe if not addressed. In the case of autoimmune diseases, the body begins to attack its own tissues, degrading them over time. If this inflammation is in the joints, such as in the case of arthritis, the cartilage begins to wear down.

In addition to autoimmune disorders, chronic inflammation can contribute to a great many illnesses, depending on how it presents, including depression, cognitive decline (such as Alzheimer's disease and other forms of dementia), age-related macular degeneration, chronic kidney disease (CKD), type 2 diabetes, certain cancers, and heart disease. These are just a few examples—chronic inflammation can underlie a great many significant threats to our bodies and minds.

Chronic inflammation can be triggered or worsened by certain lifestyle factors, such as smoking, excessive alcohol intake, drug use, obesity, insufficient sleep, chronically elevated stress levels, lowered levels of sex hormones in the body and—very notably—a poor diet. If we eat unhealthy foods, or do not get adequate levels of the nutrients our bodies need, it paves the way for chronic inflammation to thrive.

The scary thing about chronic inflammation is that if it is left unchecked, it will not likely get better on its own. Quite the contrary, it will often get a lot worse, especially if it is present for a number of years. This makes it especially important to identify and address chronic inflammation as soon as possible.

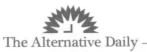

Chapter Three
Quiz: Are You Inflamed?

Chronic inflammation is the undercurrent of so many illnesses and conditions that it can be hard to pinpoint it as the source of any specific discomfort. However, there are certain warning signs of inflammation to look out for.

The following signs, symptoms and habits may indicate things other than inflammation, and do not necessarily have absolute ties to inflammation, but when trying to assess whether or not your body is inflamed, they are warning signs to watch out for, especially in combination.

- Do you find yourself feeling fatigued even when you have had sufficient sleep?
- Do you find yourself feeling depressed, anxious, lackluster or mentally foggy on a regular basis?
- Have you been experiencing lowered sex drive?
- Are you highly susceptible to any seasonal illness or bug that's going around, and/or do you feel like your immune system is not working like it should?
- Do you frequently experience allergy symptoms?
- Have you been diagnosed with an autoimmune condition, including but not limited to arthritis, asthma, Grave's disease, irritable bowel disorder (IBD) or lupus?

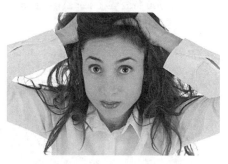

- Have you been diagnosed with metabolic syndrome?

- Have you been diagnosed with chronic kidney disease (CKD)?

- Do you have high blood pressure?

- Do you have diabetes, prediabetes or any blood sugar issues?

- Do you experience frequent digestive disturbances, including bloating, diarrhea or constipation?

- Do you experience any type of chronic pain, including neuropathy, muscle, joint or digestive pain?

- Do your joints frequently feel puffy or swollen?

- Do you feel like your joints and muscles are experiencing impaired function, or don't work as well as they used to, aside from normal age-related reasons?

- Do you have frequent skin breakouts, such as acne, eczema, psoriasis or other forms of chronic dermatitis?

- Are your eyes frequently red or bloodshot, even when they are not irritated?

- Do you habitually eat processed foods and/or fast food?

- Are there days in your week during which you do not eat fruits and vegetables?

- Do you regularly include sugar and/or wheat in your diet?

- Do you find yourself experiencing persistently high levels of stress throughout the day?

- Do you regularly get less than seven hours of sleep per night?

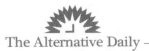

If you said yes to any of these questions, and especially if you said yes to multiple questions, it is possible that you may be experiencing chronic inflammation.

If you suspect that your body may be inflamed, your doctor can do several types of blood tests to check for markers of inflammation, such as C-reactive protein (CRP), erythrocyte sedimentation rate (ESR) and plasma viscosity (PV). However, some of these tests may be expensive, and may not test inflammation throughout your body.

The best thing to do if you suspect—or have confirmed—that you are experiencing chronic inflammation is to change your diet now. Cut out the processed foods, and stick to whole, nutritious foods from the Earth. Be sure to include an array of fruits and vegetables every day.

A natural health professional you trust may also be able to recommend some herbs and other natural remedies that may work for your individual needs.

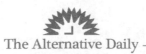

Chapter Four
Why Our Hearts Are Breaking

The human body in its healthiest state runs like a well-oiled machine. Atoms bond together to form molecules. These molecules are the makeup of cells. When cells work together, they form tissues, which in turn create organs. A group of specialized organs working together is called a system, and the combination of all of these systems together is an organism (eg., the human body), which has to fine-tune itself constantly to maintain and restore balance. This balance is called homeostasis.

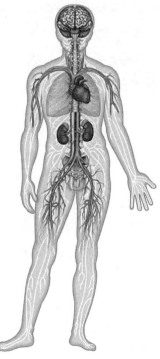

Every body, like every machine, requires constant maintenance. In the case of a machine, a trained mechanic will do routine maintenance work, make some repairs, and replace parts when they are worn and breaking. As humans, we wish our job was as simple as a quick maintenance. Unfortunately, we're a little more complicated. Our knowledge of human anatomy, of our needs and wants, increases daily, with scientists learning new facts about nutrition and health all the time.

Unfortunately, we have been force-fed information for decades about what we should eat or avoid, and this has led to a multitude of problems and diseases. We are heavier than ever before—almost 70 percent of American adults are overweight or obese. Approximately 29 million people in the U.S.

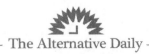

suffer from diabetes, and over 600,000 Americans die of heart disease every single year. Every day, 2,200 people die of cardiovascular diseases. 735,000 Americans suffer a heart attack every year, most of whom are men. The total number of people suffering from heart disease is a whopping 75 million!

According to the Centers for Disease Control and Prevention (CDC), heart disease is the most common cause of death in the United States in both men and women. In women, death from heart disease is more common than from all cancers combined. For instance, one in 31 American women dies of breast cancer, but one in three dies of heart disease.

Around the world, heart disease is on the rise. The world leaders for heart disease are Russia, Bulgaria, Romania, Hungary and Argentina.

Comparatively, the countries with the lowest rates of heart disease (and deaths due to heart disease) are France, Australia, Switzerland, Japan and Israel. Scientists are still stumped by these statistics, as the consumption of saturated fats and red meats have been thought to be major contributors to heart disease. Conventional wisdom in the United States dictates that the consumption of too much fat (and saturated fat in particular) is dangerous, and many medical websites recommend low-fat, high-carb diets for optimal health.

Scientists are especially surprised by France, where heart disease rates are only a quarter of those in Britain. The French are known to eat plenty of saturated fats and red meat. This phenomenon is called the "French Paradox," although we must not ignore the fact that even in these countries, with their ever-changing cultures, these diseases are also on the rise.

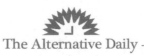

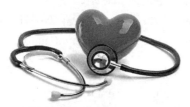

So how did we, in the United States, get here? In the 1970s, politicians had a hearing after several senators dropped dead of heart disease, and it became increasingly obvious that men in their forties and fifties were especially prone to heart disease. A Harvard University professor was heard, and he claimed that cutting the fat and increasing intake of carbohydrates would change our health and therefore increase our longevity. The first set of dietary guidelines was put into place, and America hopped on the low-fat bandwagon.

By the 90s, the low-fat craze hit an all-time high, with low-fat products practically flying off the shelves at grocery stores. We seemed to forget that the idea was originally to implement carbs like whole grains, along with more fruits and vegetables.

To Americans, fat had turned into the bad guy, and carbs (any carbs) ruled the world. Unfortunately, these carbs were usually processed (cereal, bread and pasta became staples in almost every household), and the fat was replaced by refined sugar. As a result, the average American adult now consumes over 150 pounds of sugar per year.

Sugar is not the only culprit when we look at heart disease. Your diet and lifestyle in general play a vital role. Are you severely overweight? Do you smoke? Are you always stressed out? Do you drink too much? Do you get too little exercise? Any and all of these factors can contribute to inflammation and ultimately to heart disease, but we will talk about the details of exactly what causes it, what happens, and how you can recognize it in a later part of this chapter.

It is scary to think of the numbers mentioned above. Clearly, the dietary guidelines imposed on us 40 years ago are not working, and as a result of our ever-increasing disease rates, we are more and more reliant on prescription medication to lower blood

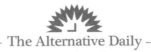

pressure and cholesterol, and to treat diseases like depression and diabetes. Rather than looking at the root cause of our problems, we are putting bandaids on them. The well-oiled machine is starting to stutter a bit, and the mechanic, overwhelmed by the sheer amount of conflicting information, sits back and does nothing.

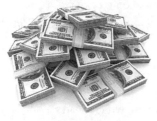

The cost of heart disease and stroke combined, according to the American Heart Association, is 312.6 billion dollars in the United States alone. This includes health-care costs and loss of income for families who are dealing with heart disease or stroke. Needless to say, these costs are still rising and will continue to do so until we implement major changes to our diets and lifestyles. Why aren't we quicker at making blanket recommendations for all Americans? This can be explained in a few ways.

1. Even though research is ruling out saturated fat and red meats as a culprit for heart disease, there is precious little research in our country on people who eat a more ancestral diet including healthy fats, meat, vegetables and fruits, and how long they live. The new information is still too fresh to make large-scale recommendations.

2. We have created a whole new problem with the way we've been treating our diseases. Millions of Americans rely on prescription medication to stay healthy, and while we can probably rule out fat and red meat as the bad guys, we'd be hard-pressed to find enough people who do not rely on some kind of medication to maintain their health and who eat a perfectly clean diet.

3. There is still too much conflicting information concerning nutrition to convince our scientists and our politicians to agree on a new direction.

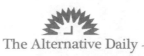

In this chapter, we will explore what heart disease is, what causes it, and talk about the difference between heart disease and cardiovascular disease. You will also learn about the cholesterol/inflammation connection and find out if cholesterol, long touted the bad guy, is truly to be feared. Finally, we'll draw the connection from your gut to your heart health and discover how everything comes full circle in our well-oiled machine. Of course, we'll also cover some practical tips on how you can lower your own risk of heart disease.

Understanding heart disease

To understand how to avoid heart disease, we have to first explore what causes it and what is happening in our body. We will also need to understand the difference between heart disease and cardiovascular disease. When we were told to replace our fats with carbohydrates, we were all too willing to oblige, and so were the food giants. Nowhere in the world are the grocery stores as loaded with colorful cereal, white bread, snack cakes and other sweet treats as in the United States. The Kellogg Company alone makes billions of dollars in sales each year of these types of products. Their message to consumers remains unchanged: eat a daily bowl of low-fat, whole-grain, sugar-laden cereal for better health.

Our relatively new understanding is that this kind of food actually makes us sicker rather than contributing to better health—and the message that we should turn to real, whole foods instead has been slow to spread throughout our population. One could argue that health is simply not lucrative enough for big corporations and the pharmaceutical industry.

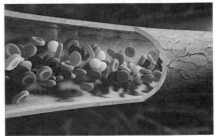

So, what is heart disease? It is an umbrella term used for a number of diseases, the most common one being coronary artery disease.

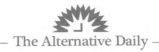

Coronary artery disease can be present for many years before you notice it. In many cases, it will lead to a heart attack (cardiovascular disease) if left untreated.

What happens when you have coronary artery disease? We thought we knew the answer to this question decades ago. It was assumed that high cholesterol, caused by fats (and especially saturated fats) was the culprit. The solution was to prescribe medication to lower cholesterol.

Dr. Dwight Lundell was a certified cardiothoracic surgeon who practiced for over 25 years and performed over 5,000 open-heart surgeries.

FACT: In 2013, Dr. Dwight Lundell, officially apologized online for decades of being wrong because he had recommended cholesterol-lowering medications and a low-fat diet.

The real cause of heart disease, according to Dr. Lundell (and a growing number of medical professionals) is inflammation. A diet high in refined carbohydrates, sugars and copious amounts of omega-6 fats (highest quantities in vegetable oils like corn oil, soybean oil and safflower oil), can cause chronic inflammation in the body.

Our bodies are not designed to process and digest these fake foods, so they wreak havoc in our arteries, causing injury to the arterial walls. According to Dr. Lundell, there is no way cholesterol would accumulate in the arteries without the presence of chronic inflammation.

But how exactly do sugary foods cause inflammation? Our bodies run on glucose. When you eat something sugary (eg., donuts), your blood sugar spikes, your pancreas releases insulin, and sugar is driven into the cells to be used for energy. All "leftovers" that cannot fit into the cells will attach to proteins in the arteries and cause injury.

Inflamed arteries look a little bit like someone scraped sandpaper over a smooth surface over and over, leaving it rough and raw. Eating high amounts of sugary treats, or pastries baked in soybean oil, day after day results in chronic inflammation.

Where do the omega-6s come in? Omega-6 fatty acids, while essential, have become more and more prevalent in our diets. While the ideal ratio of omega-6s to omega-3s varies between individuals, a ratio closer to 3:1 is considered preferable. Unfortunately, our ratios nowadays are closer to 15:1, and in some extreme cases even 30:1. This excess consumption of omega-6s causes the cell membranes to secrete a protein called cytokine, which in turn cause inflammation. Animal fats are much lower in omega-6 fatty acids than processed oils.

The buildup that occurs in the arteries is called plaque. It can take many years for plaque to build up before you notice anything. If the plaque ruptures inside an artery, this can cause a blood clot. When this happens, the oxygen-rich blood and nutrients cannot flow to the heart. This is known as a heart attack, one of the conditions that can occur when one has cardiovascular disease.

However, a heart attack doesn't have to be a death sentence. When discovered quickly, the patient can make a full recovery and live a long and happy life. It is important to understand the symptoms and warning signs of a heart attack in order to take immediate corrective action.

The most common symptom is pain in the chest. If this pain is located in the center or towards the left side, lasts more than a few minutes, and keeps returning, this may be a sign of a heart attack. Feelings of excess fullness or heartburn are also sometimes experienced.

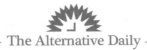

Upper body pain is another symptom. It can manifest in the neck, shoulders, jaw and chest area, all the way down to the belly button. Severe shortness of breath even when resting can also occur.

Some other symptoms may include a cold sweat, nausea and vomiting, dizziness and lightheadedness, or even feeling unusually tired, sometimes for several days. It is important to understand that heart attacks do not always start with the same symptoms.

As a matter of fact, many people are surprised to find out that they suffered from a heart attack after the fact. Regardless, if you or a loved one experience symptoms you think may be a heart attack, call 911. Minutes count when you suffer a heart attack, and an ambulance will get to you much sooner than you can get to a hospital on your own.

The big picture

We've already established that low-fat diets, high in carbs and refined sugars, do not work to lower our risk of heart disease. However, most of us have been told to do just that for as long as we can remember. It is certainly not easy to change one's mindset overnight, but doing your homework now, and understanding the bigger picture, will set you on the right track.

It may help to look back into the past a little. In the early twentieth century, pneumonia was the biggest killer of humans. It was replaced by heart disease in the 1920s when smoking spiked in the United States. Add to that the consistent growth of food giants, and the long-lasting convenience foods they introduced, and it's easy to understand why heart disease has become the number-one killer of men and women in the United States.

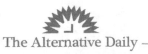

The cholesterol/inflammation connection

"Cholesterol is bad!" This has been the message for decades. Before we learned to pay attention to the LDL to HDL ratio, all we were told by doctors and the media was that a cholesterol level of over 200 was downright dangerous, and that we needed to lower our consumption of high cholesterol foods like eggs.

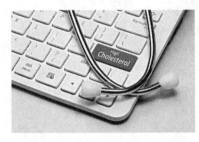

A report by Consumer Reports found that Lipitor, the most popular cholesterol lowering drug (also called a statin), was prescribed over 144 million times in 2005. This translated to over 16 billion dollars in sales. The prescriptions for Lipitor continued to soar because more and more people were diagnosed with high cholesterol, diabetes and heart disease.

What is cholesterol?

Cholesterol is a waxy substance present in every cell of our bodies, and even more prevalent in the brain (about 25 percent), where it helps to pass messages among brain cells, and helps create estrogen, progesterone, testosterone and cortisol (the stress hormone).

Cholesterol is also helpful in creating vitamin D, the sunshine vitamin, and it helps prevent gastrointestinal and respiratory illnesses. The body is capable of producing its own cholesterol, but based on your diet, it will downregulate or upregulate its own production of cholesterol.

HDL, also called "good cholesterol," is a high-density lipoprotein. It is light and fluffy. One of its jobs is to remove LDL (low-density lipoprotein), or "bad cholesterol," from

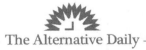

the places it doesn't belong and transport it to the liver. The ideal ratio of HDL to LDL should be 3.5 to 1, according to the American Heart Association.

Triglycerides are sometimes also measured when checking cholesterol levels, although not as often. Triglycerides are fatty acids in your bloodstream. Their numbers should be kept on the lower side, but overconsumption of sugar and grains has led to increased triglycerides in many people.

More and more doctors have become aware of the fact that it is important to look at the whole cholesterol picture, meaning HDL, LDL and triglycerides, but the majority still insist on measuring only the total number, and are quick to prescribe statins to lower cholesterol.

But is cholesterol truly the bad guy that we make it out to be?

Many doctors now believe that cholesterol is sent to a damaged blood vessel to fix it rather than to cause more damage, which leads to a higher concentration of cholesterol in damaged vessels. Numerous studies by many different scientists appear to confirm that high cholesterol is not as dangerous as we were made to believe.

A study of almost 154,000 postmenopausal women has shown that those with higher cholesterol levels actually live longer. Additionally, statins in these study participants did not manage to prevent first-time heart attacks, although the drugs did appear to be successful in preventing second heart attacks. Additionally, a study published by *The Lancet* found that statins actually increased the risk of diabetes by nine percent. Diabetes, as we've established before, is a contributor to heart disease.

As if this wasn't enough, yet more studies confirmed that in healthy women, and anyone over 69 years of age with high cholesterol, statins provided no benefits. As a

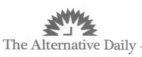

matter of fact, aggressively lowering cholesterol actually increased the occurrence of heart disease.

Of course, this takes us back to inflammation as the culprit for heart disease and ultimately heart attacks. We have covered the connection between inflammation and the consumption of sugar and high amounts of omega-6 fatty acids. The logical consequence is to make some very important changes to your diet.

Decreasing or eliminating our consumption of refined sugars—as well as foods containing refined sugars—is a great first step. Many processed foods that contain refined sugar are also high in omega-6 fatty acids. So, eliminating sugary processed food from your diet will automatically decrease your consumption of omega-6 fatty acids such as soybean and corn oil. Furthermore, when choosing fats, reach for healthy oils like olive oil, coconut oil; and even grass-fed butter, lard and beef tallow instead.

It is unfortunate that there are so few medical professionals who recommend dietary changes to lower inflammation. With a growing amount of evidence to support this recommendation, it simply makes sense to address the issue of inflammation as a cause of heart disease and to find natural ways to reduce it.

How can you help yourself? You have taken the first step by reading this book. If you haven't done so already, you can start now by changing your diet, healing your gut, reducing stress and exercising. Not smoking will also contribute to the lowering of inflammation, and your lungs will thank you for it, as you will be much better able to exercise daily.

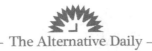

Your gut and heart disease

Reading all of this information about heart disease, cholesterol and inflammation might make your head spin, but it is nevertheless crucial to know. It may make you aware of just how important it is to maintain the health of this well-oiled machine that is your body. If one part stops working correctly, it will sooner or later impact the rest of your body, like a vicious chain reaction.

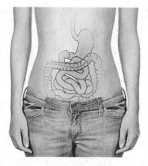

Your digestion is a north-to-south process, starting in the brain as it prepares for food. It continues down to the stomach, and on to the small and large intestines. On the way, your food is digested, broken down into valuable vitamins, minerals and other nutrients to keep you healthy. If you eat the wrong foods, your stomach can't properly digest, and this triggers the chain reaction that ultimately leads to deficiencies and diseases.

As it turns out, there's a close connection between the gut and the heart, and that a broken gut will lead to a broken heart. Conventional wisdom will have you believe that the consumption of red meat and eggs creates a chemical called trimethylamine N-oxide, or TMAO, and the theory is that TMAO increases the risk for heart disease.

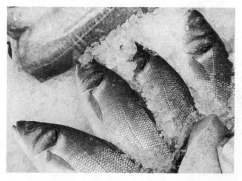

However, researchers failed to mention that things like seafood also increase TMAO levels, and we all know that scientists actually recommend the consumption of seafood. The research connecting red meat consumption to increased risk of heart disease is flawed. To get accurate information, research should also include whether the same people who eat a lot of

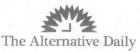

red meat tend to smoke more, drink more soda or alcohol, and exercise less, etc. None of these factors have been included in this research, so alternative practitioners are not convinced that there is any value or truth to these findings.

So, how exactly are the gut and the heart connected, and how could a broken gut cause heart disease? Firstly, your gut includes your stomach and your intestines. Small intestinal bacterial overgrowth, or SIBO, is a condition in which a large amount of bacteria is found in the small intestine. It has been linked to nutritional deficiencies, and it also causes intestinal and systemic inflammation, which could ultimately be a contributor to heart disease.

Another thing to look at is *H. pylori*, a bacteria that enters the body and starts attacking the stomach wall, which protects you from the high acidity in your stomach. This process can result in ulcers. There has been some research which found that people with *H. pylori* have a higher risk of heart disease. *H. pylori* can cause a number of problems in the body, which could lead to heart disease. Thus, it would make sense to eradicate *H. pylori*, although the truth is, most people who have *H. pylori* in their bodies won't know about it for many years.

Leaky gut (to be discussed later) may also be a contributor to heart disease. Leaky gut happens in the small intestine, where vitamins and other nutrients are absorbed through the intestinal wall. The pores of your small intestine are normally just big enough to let these nutrients through. In the case of leaky gut, inflammation causes these pores to become bigger, and larger particles of food and toxins can pass through the intestinal walls, where they will be attacked by the body. Another cause of leaky gut can be an imbalance of good versus bad bacteria in the small intestine. When the bad bacteria takes over, your gut flora will be out of balance and you can develop leaky gut.

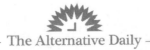

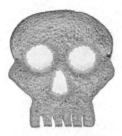

Finally, people with celiac disease are at higher risk for heart disease. Studies have found that people with celiac disease have an increased intima-media thickness of their carotid artery (a blood vessel in the neck which transports blood to the brain, face and neck), and this has been linked to an increased risk of heart disease.

According to Chris Kresser, M.S., LAc, a leader in the world of ancestral health and nutrition, it is worth taking a look at your gut microbiome. The microbiome is the population of microbes in your intestine, and about two-thirds of it is unique to each individual. We carry over four pounds of microbes in our gut, and trillions of microorganisms, with at least 1,000 species of bacteria. Changes in your gut microbiome can lead to intestinal permeability, which can cause inflammation, and as we've discussed before, inflammation is a major contributor to heart disease.

Of course, the gut is also closely tied to many other functions in the body. When in great health, your gut flora will aid in creating vitamins, absorbing minerals, removing toxins, preventing allergies and maintaining your body's natural defenses against foreign invaders and diseases. When compromised, it may play a role in weight gain, metabolic syndrome, diabetes, celiac disease and more. It is therefore crucial to maintain great gut health by eating a healthy and balanced diet. Furthermore, if you have some healing to do, it might be helpful to introduce some digestive enzymes, probiotics (many are found in whole, natural foods) and potentially some supplements. A nutritional therapy practitioner or naturopath you trust can help you get on the road to great health.

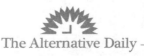

The problem with heart drugs

Statins are the most commonly prescribed drugs for lowering the risk of heart disease. Millions of Americans (one out of four adults over the age of 45) are taking statins in hopes of prolonging their lifespan, lowering their risk of heart disease and getting a handle on high cholesterol. Many studies have been conducted on the efficacy of statins; however, the results tend to lead to more questions, rather than pointing to a solution. We've mentioned earlier in this chapter that several studies found that statins are not as useful as they are made out to be.

While there are some benefits to the use of statins in certain age groups, they are certainly no wonder drug. The ever-increasing number of deaths from heart disease in the United States confirms that there is more to heart disease than lowering LDL cholesterol with statins. In a large 2010 meta-analysis of people with pre-existing heart disease who took statins for a duration of five years, a whopping 96 percent saw no benefits at all, while 1.2 percent were saved by statins, and 2.6 percent were able to prevent a heart attack. In another analysis of people without pre-existing heart disease, 98 percent saw no benefits at all, and 1.6 percent were able to prevent heart disease.

These studies also found some disturbing facts. In both cases, 10 percent of participants suffered from muscle damage due to statins, and 0.6 percent and 1.5 percent respectively developed diabetes. The Food and Drug Administration has released a report on the potential dangers of using statins. Let's look at some of the side effects that the FDA listed.

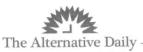

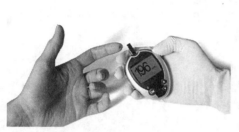

The FDA list includes the following:

Diabetes: A study of 90,000 postmenopausal women published in *The Lancet* in 2013 found a nine percent increased risk for diabetes, although the Women's Health Initiative of 2012 found in an observational study that the increased risk of using statins was actually 48 percent.

Myopathy: Muscle damage can occur in patients taking statins, especially in connection with other drugs. Muscle pain is one of the most common side effects of statin use, and this can be mild or very severe. If you experience muscle pain while taking statins, please talk to your doctor.

Liver damage: Statins work in the liver to lower the production of cholesterol. The FDA recommends getting liver enzymes tested before patients start taking statins. During treatment, it is advisable to test occasionally. Some scientists downplay the risks of liver damage from statins, and say that the benefits outweigh the risks. The symptoms of liver damage can be fatigue, pain in the upper right abdomen, pain between the shoulder blades, dark urine, and loss of appetite. See a doctor immediately if you have any of these symptoms.

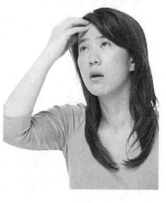

Memory loss: This can occur in all patients, male or female, and regardless of age. Patients have described feeling fuzzy and having "senior moments." It is strongly suggested to see your doctor if you experience memory loss while taking statins.

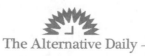

We need to pay attention to short-term side effects when treating any of our health issues as they can have a pretty substantial impact on our long term health, especially when it comes to your liver. Your liver is your body's powerhouse and detox factory, and it performs over 300 functions.

In over 900 studies of statin drugs, a much longer list of side effects has been found. These findings were published in the *American Journal of Cardiovascular Drugs*.

These side effects include the following:

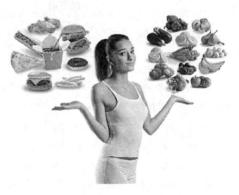

- Neuropathy

- Anemia

- Frequent fevers

- Acidosis

- Cataracts

- Sexual dysfunction

- Cognitive loss

- Increase in cancer risk

- Pancreatic dysfunction

- Hepatic (liver) dysfunction (due to the effect of statins on the liver)

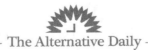

What you can do right now to reduce your risk

By following the recommendations below, you will not only lower your risk of heart disease, you will also become healthier, and increase your chances of staying healthy.

Limit or eliminate your consumption of refined sugar. Your body is perfectly capable of using real food to create glucose. Your body doesn't recognize sugar as food, and you won't recognize when you've had enough. Therefore, you are much more likely to overeat sugar and sugary foods. Best to stay away!

Eat plenty of vegetables and fruit. Spinach, avocados, broccoli, blueberries, citrus fruits and tomatoes are just a few examples to choose from. Pay attention to how you feel, certain vegetables and fruits while healthy for many, may actually not be your friend. As a general guideline, if it makes you feel worse when you consume it, don't.

Enjoy grass-fed meat and cold-water fatty fish. The fats and nutrients in fish and grass-fed meat are plentiful, and will fill you up much quicker than any sugary treat.

Choose healthy fats. These include extra virgin olive oil, unrefined coconut oil, grass-fed butter, natural lard, beef tallow, ghee and raw nuts.

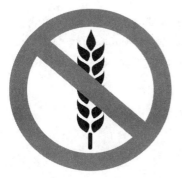

Avoid eating processed and glutenous grains. Many grains, especially those that contain gluten, can have an inflammatory effect on the body. If you are confused about the grain issue, or you're searching for natural, gluten-free grains that you can work into your healthy diet, we recommend having a conversation with a nutritionist or natural health professional you trust to find out which grains can work for you—and which to avoid.

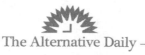

By making these adjustments to your diet, you will help to balance your insulin levels, and therefore improve your body's ability to handle sugar. You will also greatly reduce inflammation in your body.

Legumes should be soaked and sprouted to make them more digestible. The soaking of legumes and grains removes anti-nutrients like phytates, which can damage the gut. While phytates are necessary for good health, over-consumption leads to problems like inflammation and leaky gut.

Making dietary changes is a great start—probably the most important one. However, you may also benefit from proper supplementation, especially if you are just getting started on your journey to better health. Years, and sometimes decades, of yo-yo dieting can deplete you of important vitamins and other nutrients. For this reason, certain supplements can be helpful in healing your gut.

Probiotics. Probiotics are a great way to heal your gut flora, and they are present in naturally fermented foods like sauerkraut and kimchi, raw kefir and kombucha. If you (or a nutritional professional of your choice) feel you need a little extra support, you'll find probiotics in the health food section of your grocery store. They are usually cooled and need to be stored in your refrigerator.

Magnesium. This mineral is needed for over 300 biochemical functions in your body, and many people are deficient in magnesium without knowing it. Magnesium has been linked to a reduced risk of sudden cardiac death. If taken at night, it can help you fall asleep and stay asleep longer.

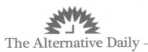

Fermented cod liver oil (FCLO). Increase your amount of omega-3 fatty acids by taking FCLO on a daily basis. You don't need to swallow the oil, as it also comes in pills and tablets. It may be advisable to do this at night to avoid the unpleasant fishy burps.

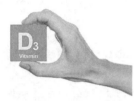

Vitamin D3. Almost all people in the northern United States are deficient in vitamin D. If you cannot get out into the sun daily, consider taking a vitamin D supplement. Some studies have found that low levels of vitamin D carry an increased risk of heart disease.

When opting for nutritional supplements, be sure to purchase a reputable brand you trust, as the ingredients are of much better quality, and no unnecessary fillers are used. Do your research thoroughly, or ask a health provider you trust for a recommendation, as many imposters lurk on the shelves.

Next to diet, **sleep** should be your top priority. People who get around eight hours of sleep per night function better and for longer periods during the day. Adequate sleep also helps regulate insulin levels and is associated with less weight gain. Decreased amounts of sleep are linked to an increased risk for diabetes, which is a contributor to heart disease. If you have trouble sleeping, try to understand why so that you can make the necessary changes towards a healthy sleep cycle.

The use of beta blockers can inhibit the production of melatonin and keep you from falling asleep. Supplementation may be in order (as always, it is best to talk to a health professional you trust before going this route). Stop using technology before going to bed, as phones and computer screens simulate daylight and will also prevent the production of melatonin. Developing and sticking to a nightly routine will help you calm down and relax.

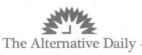

Stop smoking. According to the CDC, smoking is linked to increased risk of heart disease, stroke and lung cancer. It damages blood vessels, and the narrowing of blood vessels is linked to heart disease. The CDC also lists a number of other cancers that can be caused by cigarette smoking. If you smoke, it's time to quit—for the sake of your overall health.

Exercise. Exercising daily (from moderate to vigorous) helps with weight loss, weight maintenance, balancing blood pressure, lowering LDL cholesterol, building muscle, improving mood and increasing stamina. Additionally, it is important to stand and walk often to break up any time you spend sitting. Try to go for a walk daily, and frequently stand up from your chair or couch.

Meditate. Meditation has experienced a great boom in the Western world lately, although it has been around for thousands of years. Meditation is widely used for stress management. Stress is a contributing factor to heart disease. In a recent randomized trial, results showed that daily meditation decreased the risk of death from stroke, heart attack and other causes by 48 percent. Meditation doesn't have to be an hour-long event. Even 15 minutes a day can help you reduce stress.

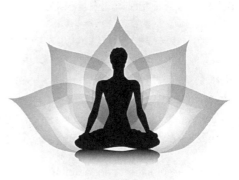

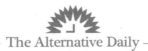

Chapter Five
The Sugar Shack: The Rise of Diabetes

Diabetes rates have been rising around the globe, and the number of deaths directly caused by diabetes has passed one and a half million per year, according to statistics compiled by the World Health Organization (WHO). The Global Status Report on Noncommunicable Diseases 2012, published by the WHO, states, "In 2014 the global prevalence of diabetes was estimated to be 9 percent among adults aged 18+ years." The rise of diabetes around the world can be attributed to several factors, including obesity, poor food choices, and a sedentary lifestyle.

Americans have also experienced a large number of diabetes diagnoses, mainly due to poor diet and the rising prevalence of obesity in the United States. According to the American Diabetes Association, approximately 29 million Americans have diabetes—that's about 9.3 percent of the population. The CDC has also found that there are approximately eight million Americans undiagnosed. According to 2014 research published in *The Journal of the American Medical Association (JAMA)*, 34.9 percent of adults are obese. The death toll from diabetes also continues to rise in America, killing approximately 70,000 every year. Diabetes ranks seventh on the CDC's "leading causes of death."

The connection between obesity, inflammation, and diabetes has a long history, and research is beginning to uncover a variety of links between diabetes and inflammation. Recent research discusses the role of inflammation and bacteria in the body, specifically in the stomach, which puts people at higher risk for diabetes. Most of these toxic changes happen in the fat cells of the stomach, and this may be the link between obesity and diabetes, specifically type 2 diabetes.

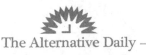

A 2005 study published in *The Journal of Clinical Investigation* discusses, "the molecular and cellular underpinnings of obesity-induced inflammation and the signaling pathways at the intersection of metabolism and inflammation that contribute to diabetes." Current research has been investigating the normal inflammatory response in our bodies and the role of metabolic support for maintaining a natural, healthy inflammatory response.

Inflammatory cytokines are currently seen as one of the main culprits behind the body's inflammatory response, and are linked to the onset of type 2 diabetes. Inflammatory cytokines are also aggravated by oxidative stress - a condition that occurs when free radicals are out of control, which is primarily caused by environmental stresses, including what foods we consume (sugar heavily contributes to oxidative stress, vegetables have an antioxidant effect).

The grouping of inflammatory cytokines is one aspect of the inflammatory response of the body. A higher inflammatory response caused by a flood of grouped inflammatory cytokines can have severe consequences. One of these is type 2 diabetes, which may also cause more than a handful of other serious health conditions. A 2003 study published in the journal *Diabetes* states, "Our data suggest that the pattern of inflammatory cytokines is important in the pathogenesis of type 2 diabetes."

According to recent research, one in three Americans currently has prediabetes, and by 2025, one in five Americans will have diabetes. Still not alarmed? Research estimates also show that by 2050, one in three Americans will have diabetes, which will equate to well over 100 million people. Along with health issues, the economic issues associated with diabetes in America are also horrific—an estimated 245 billion dollars in medical costs and lost wages!

It is essential to know if you are at risk for diabetes, and if you are, it's important to understand the steps you need to take to prevent yourself from becoming another

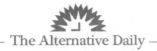

diabetes statistic in the very near future. Understanding the role of inflammation, the metabolic response, and the immune system as it relates to diabetes—specifically type 2 diabetes—is paramount. Changes in diet and obtaining the knowledge you need is the first step to a healthy, diabetes-free future.

Are you at risk?

Many Americans are at risk for diabetes, and continue to be unaware of the dangers that await them if they do not take action immediately. Prediabetics often have higher blood sugar than normal, but let's be honest, how often do you check your blood sugar levels?

According to the CDC, over 86 million adults are prediabetic. This means that over an additional quarter of the population is at risk for developing type 2 diabetes. The CDC also states that 15 to 30 percent of all prediabetics will develop type 2 diabetes within five years. Your knowledge concerning diabetes is key, and without it, you may be at severe risk.

Being at risk for diabetes may also mean you are at risk for other serious health conditions that will affect your entire life. If you understand what is going on in your body, you will have a better understanding of the whole picture, allowing you to really examine the health choices you are making on a daily basis.

Gaining the essential knowledge you need to prevent and fight diabetes begins with you. Are you prediabetic? What is your lifestyle like? Are you making healthy choices day in and day out? The road to a healthier and happier you starts with these questions, and taking a good, long, hard look at your lifestyle is the first step to enjoying more years, free of illness and the stress associated with it.

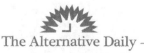

Diabetes quiz

If you don't think diabetes is a serious health issue, it is important to understand the very cold, hard facts. Sure, managing diabetes can be simple for some, and lifestyle changes may prevent or slow future complications associated with diabetes. However, diabetes remains a serious, life-shattering illness with an extremely high mortality rate. The American Diabetes Association states, "Two out of three people with diabetes die from heart disease or stroke." In fact, diabetes kills more Americans per year than breast cancer and AIDS.

The questions in this diabetes quiz have been adapted from tests provided by the American Diabetes Association and the Centers for Disease Control and Prevention. They can be used as starting points in a conversation between you and your doctor, to help determine your prediabetes and diabetes risk. They can also help you isolate some lifestyle factors that may be contributing to your risk.

Are you male or female?

This factor is important because research has shown men to be less willing to have regular checkups with a doctor.

If female, have you given birth to a baby weighing more than nine pounds?

Gestational diabetes is a concern for women.

Do you have a family member with diabetes?

Having a relative with diabetes may contribute to your risk for developing type 2 diabetes.

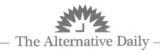

Have you ever been diagnosed with hypertension (high blood pressure)?

Hypertension puts you at risk for diabetes.

What is your age range (less than 40, 40–49, 50–59, 60 or older)?

Age has been found to be a factor in developing diabetes.

What is your race / ethnicity?

Certain races and ethnicities are more at risk than others.

Are you physically active?

Your level of physical activity can be a factor in whether or not you develop diabetes.

What is your body mass index (BMI)?

Your body mass index is important in understanding your height and weight proportions, which, as with obesity, can directly affect your chance of developing diabetes.

The above questions outline some of the more general risk factors associated with developing type 2 diabetes. If you understand these risk factors (the ones that are modifiable) and take the necessary preventative steps, you are less likely to develop diabetes.

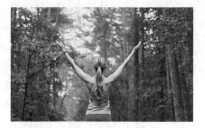

However, ignoring these factors may put you at risk for becoming one of over 80 million Americans who are prediabetic.

Education about diabetes has become one of the most important issues in the United States, since many Americans are classified as obese. The American Medical

INFLAMMATION ERASED:

NATURALLY FIGHT & REVERSE DAMAGING INFLAMMATORY EFFECTS IN YOUR BODY

Association has partnered with the CDC and developed a plan to educate, screen, test and begin to beat back prediabetes and diabetes.

These organizations have developed important screening procedures and tests for diabetes. According to this statement:

"The Centers for Disease Control and Prevention (CDC) and the American Medical Association (AMA) are sounding an alarm about prediabetes because a national effort—by everyone from physicians to employers to patients to community organizations—is required to prevent type 2 diabetes in the United States. In addition to focusing on the person with prediabetes or diabetes, we also must engage the systems and communities where people live, work and play. We can all Act – Today."

Just as it's important for you to understand your risk for diabetes, gaining key knowledge about inflammation may also save your life. Research has shown inflammation to be linked to diabetes, and it is essential for your health to understand the risk factors associated with inflammation as well. In fact, two of the most beneficial lifestyle changes for diabetes, fitness and diet, are also associated with preventing inflammation.

One of the most common health risks associated with diabetes is obesity, and obesity is also a key factor when it comes to inflammatory disease. A 2006 study published in *European Cytokine Network* states, "Obesity corresponds to a subclinical inflammatory condition that promotes the production of pro-inflammatory factors involved in the pathogenesis of insulin resistance." Many of the health questions related to diabetes may also correspond with inflammatory disease, and obtaining knowledge about both is essential to your health and wellness.

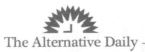

Understanding type 1 diabetes (hypoglycemia)

Type 1 diabetes is more commonly diagnosed in children and adolescents, and was once known as juvenile diabetes. According to the American Diabetes Association, only five percent of all people living with diabetes have type 1 diabetes. In order to understand type 1 diabetes, we must understand the function of insulin. Insulin is a key

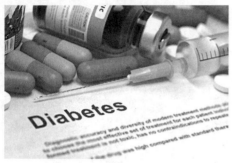

hormone created in the pancreas, needed for your body to convert nutrients and foods like sugar and starch into energy. In the case of type 1 diabetes, the body fails to produce the essential insulin needed for healthy function. Currently, there are no known prevention strategies for type 1 diabetes, and the cause is yet to be discovered.

A few common warnings that may occur are polyuria (large quantities of diluted urine, or urinating too often), polydipsia (extreme thirst), weight loss and extreme vision changes. Living with type 1 diabetes is manageable by adopting a lifestyle based around blood glucose management, daily insulin injection, diet, exercise and controlling stress levels. Type 1 diabetes is usually diagnosed early in a person's life, and the individual must learn the lifestyle choices needed for maintaining a healthy and happy life.

Type 1 diabetes does carry many serious health risks and illnesses, associated with a lifetime of insulin control and injection. Statistics compiled by the Juvenile Diabetes Research Foundation (JDRF) state that over 1.25 million American are living with type 1 diabetes, and 40,000 people are diagnosed with the disease each year. JDRF also reports that people with type 1 diabetes have a 13 year shorter life expectancy.

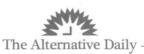

Understanding type 2 diabetes (hyperglycemia)

Type 2 diabetes accounts for the other 95 percent of diabetes diagnoses, and is a very serious illness. However, it is preventable and reversible in many cases. Type 2 diabetes is also known as "non-insulin dependent diabetes," as it usually develops in the later stages of life (the incidence of type 2 diabetes in youth has seen an alarming increase in modern times). Many cases of type 2 diabetes can be attributed to personal choices made by individuals concerning their health. The World Health Organization (WHO) suggests that type 2 diabetes, "is largely the result of excess body weight and physical inactivity."

People who are diagnosed with type 2 diabetes have above normal blood glucose levels, and the insulin their bodies produce is used ineffectively. In prediabetes, the pancreas overworks itself to create insulin levels to balance blood glucose. However, the pancreas eventually fails to keep up and more serious health issues arise.

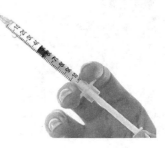

The early signs of type 2 diabetes are often overlooked unless precautionary steps, tests and knowledge of the disease are obtained. Many people do not fully understand the effect type 2 diabetes has on the body. Not knowing if you are at risk for type 2 diabetes, or having type 2 diabetes without diagnosis, causes glucose levels to build, thus potentially leading to serious health conditions like heart, kidney, vision and neurological failure.

Obesity-related type 2 diabetes cases are increasing dramatically in the United States, as many Americans continue to ignore healthy dietary choices which could greatly reduce their risk.

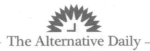

Obesity and the large amount of fat cells associated with obesity plays a large role in inflammation. Recent research has focused on inflammation as a link between obesity and type 2 diabetes. Inflammation, obesity and type 2 diabetes are also associated with metabolic syndrome, a cluster, or "perfect storm," of health issues which may lead to higher blood pressure, increased blood sugar and excess fat around the waist area. A 2014 study published in *Diabetes Research and Clinical Practice* discusses the physiological links between these illnesses. The authors state, "Systemic inflammatory markers are risk factors for the development of type 2 diabetes and its macrovascular complications."

Understanding gestational diabetes

Gestational diabetes is an in-between type of diabetes which occurs during some pregnancies. Women who develop gestational diabetes during pregnancy experience high blood glucose levels, however, these levels are still too low to qualify for a diagnosis of type 2 diabetes. Gestational diabetes puts women at serious risk for complications during their pregnancy and delivery. Women who develop gestational diabetes are also at risk for developing type 2 diabetes after their pregnancy.

The signs and symptoms of gestational diabetes are often not found until women discuss their risk with their doctors during pregnancy. This conversation usually occurs around the 24th week of pregnancy. A 2014 study published in the CDC's "Preventing Chronic Disease" discusses the prevalence of gestational diabetes. The research found, "GDM prevalence is as high as 9.2 percent."

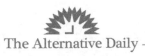

Diabetic domino effect

Developing any type of diabetes is a life-changing event. This is especially true in the case of type 2 diabetes. Prediabetes spurs a domino effect that can lead to type 2 diabetes and other serious health problems. Inflammation is also a part of the diabetic domino effect, a causal and continual issue which may put your body on a deadly downward spiral.

There are numerous studies and recent research publications discussing the development of inflammatory issues and the link between inflammation and diabetes. A 2015 study published in the *British Journal of Nutrition* suggests, "an unresolved inflammatory response is likely to be involved from the early stages of disease development." In the multiple tipping points associated with developing type 2 diabetes, inflammation remains at the core in many ways, including its role in obesity-related diabetes diagnoses.

As previously discussed, cytokines, specifically clustered cytokines, have a role to play in inflammation in regards to metabolic syndrome, type 2 diabetes and immune function. The above-mentioned study also states, "In particular cytokines in the fasting state… are recognised as an insensitive and highly variable index of tissue inflammation." A clear view of the diabetic domino effect can be traced from the several risk factors associated with diabetes, including health issues related to inflammatory disease.

Where does diabetes begin, and where does it lead you? In the case of type 2 diabetes, it begins with lifestyle choices! As we mentioned, type 2 diabetes makes up approximately 95 percent of all diabetes cases, and this serious disease involves lifestyle choices made long before you are actually diagnosed.

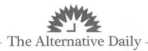

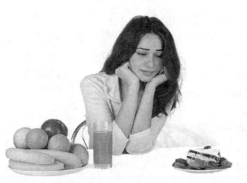

An unhealthy diet and lack of activity often leads to becoming overweight or obese. With obesity on the rise, it is no wonder the future looks grim. Being overweight is the primary risk factor for developing type 2 diabetes, and this is where it begins. There are other risk factors, however, none are as evident as obesity, or "diabesity." Diabesity is a term for a metabolic dysfunction combining several risk factors ranging from high blood sugar, high blood pressure, abdominal obesity and systemic inflammation. People with these symptoms of diabesity may not be diagnosed with type 2 diabetes yet, but they are without a doubt prediabetic.

Recent research suggests that over one billion people in the world suffer from diabesity, with 100 million Americans on the top of the list. It has been found that diabesity will continue to rise, and the number of people who will develop diabesity, prediabetes, or type 2 diabetes is astounding. It is also suggested that diabesity and the risk factors associated with it may be the number one killer in the world.

How do you protect yourself from diabesity, you ask? The answer is simple: gear your lifestyle towards health. Choose nutritious, whole foods which naturally manage your weight, and perform some type of physical activity at least three times a week.

A 2013 study published in *PLoS One* states, "Prevalence of obesity, diabetes and accompanying disturbances has increased globally, reaching epidemic levels in adults, adolescents, and even children. To prevent the further spread of this epidemic, identifying early risk factors is urgently needed to develop appropriate prevention strategies."

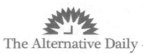

Diabesity is, in essence, a matter of choice, and that choice is yours. Making healthier lifestyle choices, including diet and exercise, and understanding diabesity is the first step in prevention. With this understanding and these healthier choices you eliminate the primary forerunner of the diabetic domino effect and increase your chances of living a longer, healthier and happier life without the scourge of diabetes setting in.

The research performed on inflammation, diabesity, prediabetes and type 2 diabetes paints a clear picture of their intertwined nature. Diabetes can lead to inflammation, and inflammation can lead to diabetes, plain and simple.

Inflammation may well be the first domino in the diabetes domino effect. A 2013 study published in the *Journal of Leukocyte Biology* discusses inflammation and the macrophages which attack the pancreas causing insulin resistance, and later, diabetes. The research findings state, "The innate immunity matures in a diabetes-dependent manner from an initial proinflammatory toward a profibrotic phenotype, supporting the concept that T2D [type 2 diabetes] is an inflammatory disease."

Inflammation begins to wreak havoc on the pancreas, causing insulin resistance, prediabetes and then type 2 diabetes may be diagnosed. Soon, without major lifestyle changes, you may begin to experience other illnesses, and possible very serious diseases. Heart disease, nerve damage (neuropathy), liver damage, kidney disease (nephropathy), visual impairment, skin problems, Alzheimer's disease, stroke and many more illnesses are among the serious health conditions type 2 diabetes may lead to.

The diabetic domino effect can be avoided, and you can fight inflammation and prevent yourself from developing diabetes by gaining knowledge and evaluating your current lifestyle. Are you taking the necessary steps to fight inflammation and diabetes?

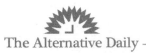

What is HbA1C? You need to know!

Glycated haemoglobin, or HbA1C, occurs when red blood cell proteins combine with glucose in the blood, which in turn becomes glycated. This glycated haemoglobin is an essential part of diabetes testing. Testing for HbA1C allows doctors to gauge your average blood sugar levels over a period of time, often weeks or months.

Why is this important? This essential blood test will give you a more accurate picture of how well your diabetes is being managed over time. The standard finger prick, which checks your immediate blood sugar levels, is often not an accurate picture. Not knowing your blood sugar patterns over time can make complications from diabetes more prevalent.

The HbA1C test is essential even for individuals who do not have diabetes, as well as for those who have already been diagnosed with diabetes. People with diabetes should have this test done often— every 3 months—to keep a close eye on their diabetes management. However, most doctors recommend this test only twice 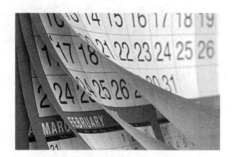 a year. The National Institute of Diabetes and Digestive and Kidney Diseases has outlined normal percentages, and stresses the importance of the HbA1C test. The normal reading for the HbA1C blood test is in the range from 4.0 to 5.6 percent. A reading in the range from 5.7 to 6.4 percent representing prediabetes, and a reading of 6.5 percent or more representing fully developed diabetes.

This test is also an essential marker for prediabetic diagnoses. The number of Americans who are prediabetic is staggering, especially since the diabetic domino effect may lead to some very frightening medical problems. The HbA1C test can help

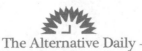

doctors diagnose more of the over 86 million people who may be prediabetic, according to the CDC. The HbA1C test can make a huge impact on early detection, allowing you a fighting chance to prevent a full diabetic diagnosis.

The National Institute of Diabetes and Digestive and Kidney Diseases also suggests, "Because the A1C test does not require fasting and blood can be drawn for the test at any time of day, experts are hoping its convenience will allow more people to get tested—thus, decreasing the number of people with undiagnosed diabetes." If people took a more active role in diabetes prevention, this test could save millions of lives.

Another positive aspect of this essential blood test is the "skinny diabetic" factor. Not all people who have diabetes, or prediabetes, are overweight. One major misconception is that only obese people get diabetes, and that if you are skinny and in relatively good shape, your risk for developing type 2 diabetes is nonexistent.

Unfortunately, this "skinny" thinking is a diabetes myth which could actually cause someone to miss the prediabetic warning signs and fall down the type 2 diabetes rabbit hole. If you are skinny and are having more than a couple of the type 2 diabetes symptoms outlined by the CDC—excessive thirst, frequent urination, weight loss, hunger, numbness in hands and feet, vision changes, dry skin and general weakness and malaise—you should look into getting the HbA1C test.

The odds may be stacked against those with a genetic predisposition for developing type 2 diabetes. It is estimated that one in three people who currently have type 2 diabetes is undiagnosed, therefore HbA1C testing is essential. Skinny, average, overweight or obese, if you have any family members with diabetes, or if you are experiencing any diabetic symptoms, it is important to get the glycated haemoglobin test and discuss your health concerns with your doctor.

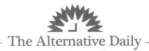

Recent research has uncovered further contributing factors to a diabetes diagnosis: genetics, fatty liver, inflammation, autoimmunity and stress are all factors found in the development of diabetes, whether you are skinny or obese, genetically predisposed or physically inactive. Interestingly enough, inflammation is a huge factor in "skinny diabetes," causing the same inflammatory cytokines to hinder insulin production.

A 2015 study published in the *Indian Journal of Endocrinology and Metabolism* discusses the differences in body composition between Asian-Indians and Caucasians, suggesting that type 2 diabetes is just as prevalent in skinny people. The study states, "In East-Asians, even with slightest instability and vulnerability in canalization of beta cell, with a concomitant decrease in insulin secretion can easily promote diabetogenesis." The skinny diabetic factor may not be the most seen or even understood aspect of diabetes, however, it may contribute to the statistics. The HbA1C test can assist health organizations around the globe to get a more accurate picture of diabetes, while giving people the life-saving results they need in order to manage diabetes that they might have otherwise not known about.

Diabetic drug dangers

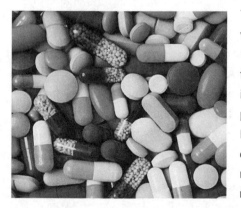

Treating diabetes with drugs may pose a wide variety of dangers. In the case of type 1 diabetes, there may be some implications for drugs, since this specific type of diabetes is an autoimmune disease in which insulin production from the pancreas is nonexistent. However, as we have mentioned, 95 percent of cases are type 2 diabetes that are often related to lifestyle choices, and these may be managed differently.

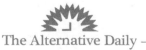

In most cases of type 2 diabetes, unhealthy choices created the diabetic domino effect, and oftentimes, management in these cases can be most effective through positive lifestyle choices. However, some cases are genetic, and treatment options may differ. We will discuss the type 2 diabetes cases that are lifestyle-induced, caused by inflammation, obesity, diabesity and other risk factors.

Utilizing drugs to treat type 2 diabetes may be quite harmful, and some research has found that these drugs may actually kill you. The drugs used to treat type 2 diabetes are aimed at lowering blood sugar levels. This practice has been subject to much scrutiny, and recent research has found that attempting to lower blood sugar levels, whether effective or not, could cause serious cardiac problems.

A 2011 study published in the *British Medical Journal* discusses the dangers involved in lowering blood sugar levels via prescribed medications. The study aimed to compile evidence relating to the cardiovascular-related mortality and overall death rates associated with diabetic drugs. The study found a noneffective percentage difference between the blood sugar lowering effects of these drugs and cardiovascular-related deaths. The study suggests, "The overall results of this meta-analysis show limited benefits of intensive glucose lowering treatment on all cause mortality and deaths from cardiovascular causes."

One of the most dangerous drugs used to treat diabetes was Avandia, also known in the pharmaceutical market as rosiglitazone. Avandia was, in a sense, an insulin sensitivity drug which made diabetics more sensitive to the natural insulin their bodies produced. Patients were prescribed Avandia in hopes of regulating their blood sugar levels, however, the body's organs were directly affected by this drug.

A 2007 study published in the *New England Journal of Medicine* compiled various studies and research from Avandia clinical trials via the Food and Drug Administration (FDA) and found some shocking results. The study found that "Rosiglitazone was

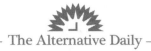

associated with a significant increase in the risk of myocardial infarction and with an increase in the risk of death from cardiovascular causes that had borderline significance." The mean baseline for the study consisted of diabetic cases with an 8.2 percent average mark given by the HbA1C glycated haemoglobin test.

Avandia proved to be extremely dangerous for those with type 2 diabetes, and offered up a plethora of severe side effects to those taking the drug. Stroke, heart failure and other cardiovascular health issues have been recorded in approximately 80,000 diabetics who took Avandia to manage their blood sugar levels.

The Food and Drug Administration (FDA) and European Medicines Agency have taken steps to eliminate drugs like Avandia until further trials and research can approve their safe use. Other dangerous diabetes drugs include Actos (pioglitazone) and Glucophage (metformin), which are at the forefront of research scrutinizing their effectiveness and safety. There have also been an increasing number of lawsuits associated with the drugs used to manage and treat diabetes.

As we've suggested, type 2 diabetes can often be managed through lifestyle changes and choices geared towards health. Whether you are prediabetic, suffer from diabesity or have been diagnosed with diabetes—and even if you are currently within an acceptable HbA1C percentage—consuming a healthy, whole-food diet combined with an active lifestyle will help you to manage or prevent diabetes.

The American Diabetes Association suggests, "Eating well-balanced meals is an essential part of taking better care of yourself and managing diabetes. So is regular physical activity, which is especially important for people with diabetes and those at risk for diabetes. Balancing what you eat and your physical activity are key to managing diabetes."

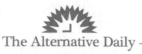

Managing blood sugar is important for health in people with diabetes, however, managing diabetes should also be approached from the "ground up." The underlying causes of any disease or illness need to be addressed in order to restore health to the body. Currently, medicine embodies a more "treat the symptoms and not the cause" philosophy, which alleviates acute problems, but leaves the chronic health issues lurking beneath. Research has found diabetes to be caused by insulin secretion and poor leptin signaling. These two issues should be at the heart of the management strategy for all diabetes patients.

Leptin is often referred to as the "fat hormone," although this term is actually contradictory to the physiological role of leptin in the body. Leptin is a protein which tells your brain whether your energy stores are sufficient or unbalanced. When your brain is satisfied with the leptin levels in your body, you will begin burning energy in a normal way. If your leptin is unbalanced and your brain senses this imbalance, your brain stimulates your vagus nerve and you become hungry. Your body essentially goes into a state of leptin deficiency, which research has shown to be a factor in obesity. A 1998 study published in *Nature* states, "In humans, leptin deficiency due to a mutation in the leptin gene is associated with early-onset obesity."

Inflammation, as discussed previously, has been researched diligently as a factor in both obesity and diabetes. Inflammation is also directly linked to your body's leptin levels. Chronic inflammation has been found to cause negative signaling to your brain, and may lead to leptin, insulin and cortisol resistance. "Leptin and Inflammation" is a study published in 2008 in *HHS Author Manuscripts*. This study discusses the intimate relationship that leptin and inflammation share.

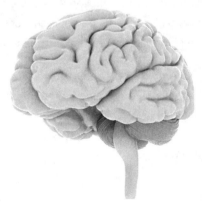

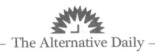

The Alternative Daily

"Several studies have implicated leptin in the pathogenesis of chronic inflammation, and the elevated circulating leptin levels in obesity appear to contribute to the low-grade inflammatory background which makes obese individuals more susceptible to increased risk of developing cardiovascular diseases, type II diabetes, or degenerative disease including autoimmunity and cancer."

Diabetes should be addressed from its root cause. Research suggests that the underlying factors in diabetes are inflammation and the chemical imbalances in your body that create resistance to insulin and leptin. Managing diabetes is really about managing the causes of inflammation, as well as managing obesity through healthy lifestyle choices. Treating the disease with a wide array of pharmaceutical drugs is not an effective course of action because these drugs do nothing to address the root issues, and as mentioned, research has found that they may do more harm than good. Obtaining more knowledge about inflammation and getting rid of the first few dominos in the diabetic domino effect is very important in your battle against diabetes and inflammation.

Prevention and healthy management of diabetes begins today

Preventing and managing diabetes, specifically type 2 diabetes, begins with looking at your lifestyle. Your diet and level of physical activity play a major role in type 2 diabetes management and prevention. According to the Diabetes Prevention Program (DPP), research compiled by the National Institute of Diabetes and Digestive and Kidney Diseases states, "Type 2 diabetes is a disorder that affects the way the body uses digested food for growth and energy." Eating whole, nutritious foods, along with staying active, are key to better digestion and optimal energy use by the body.

The CDC discusses how lifestyle changes can greatly decrease your risk for developing prediabetes, diabesity, and type 2 diabetes, and states that by making two lifestyle changes, diet and exercise, you can likely add more years to your life.

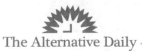

Diet is an extremely important aspect of diabetes prevention and control, with recent research focusing on eating more whole, nutritious foods instead of medication to lower blood sugar levels. Science has found that sticking to natural foods will increase your health, help control your weight, and battle the cytokines associated with inflammation. The CDC states, "Learning how to eat right is an important part of controlling your diabetes."

Skipping specific foods, those which damage the body, will also help prevent or manage prediabetes, diabetes and inflammation. The most important thing you can do for your diet is to cut out processed foods. These "fake foods" lend little-to-no nutritional value to your body, and their chemical-ridden nature can do a lot of harm. Also, avoiding sugar is key, as sugar is highly inflammatory. Anything deep-fried should also be off the menu. Glutenous grains may also cause both inflammation and weight gain. When it comes to fats, stick to unprocessed, natural oils such as coconut oil, extra virgin olive oil and grass-fed butter. In moderation, these healthy fats can actually boost healthy weight loss.

Don't worry, there are still a huge variety of delicious foods to choose from! The list of whole foods rich in nutritional goodness and anti-inflammatory potency is almost endless. Eating more fiber is recommended by the CDC for preventing and managing diabetes. High-fiber superfoods you can add to your daily menu include gluten-free whole grains like steel-cut oats and quinoa, as well as vegetables like artichokes, brussels sprouts, leafy greens and broccoli. Beans are also high-fiber diabetes-fighters, with lentils and black beans containing 15 grams of fiber per cup.

Eating fruit is also a wonderful way to prevent and manage diabetes and inflammation. Fruits with the skin left on are the best. Some great choices include pears, apples, raspberries and blackberries. Raspberries and blackberries are excellent fruits for preventing any illness, since they are well known for their high antioxidant content and

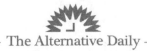

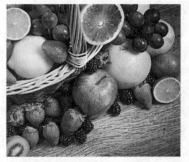

free-radical-fighting abilities. A 2014 study published in the *Journal of Agriculture and Food Chemistry* suggests, "Fruits, such as berries, contain polyphenol compounds purported to have anti-inflammatory activity in humans." Just remember, it is best to eat your fruit fresh, whole, in moderation and preferably early in the day. It is also important to choose organically grown fruits whenever possible.

On that note, certain fruits and vegetables if grown conventionally (non-organically) pose a higher risk while some conventionally grown ones might be considered safer. The Environmental Working Group produces a current list of what they refer to as "The Dirty Dozen", those fruits and vegetables that should be purchased organically, as well as the "Clean 15", the ones where conventionally grown is a safer option.

Note: If you have been diagnosed with prediabetes or diabetes, you may need to stay away from fruits with a higher sugar content, such as bananas and other tropical fruits. In some cases, these can be acceptable in moderation, but talk to your health professional just to be sure if you have received a diabetes-related diagnosis.

Another important step when remaking your diet is to eat healthy portion sizes, especially when eating starchy foods, such as potatoes and gluten-free grains. The National Institute of Diabetes and Digestive and Kidney Diseases has outlined a few great tips to help you with portion sizes: use smaller dishes, plates and bowls; eat meals regularly; eat slowly; and eat food mindfully. Being mindful of food in general will help you to really evaluate what you're putting into your body, and its nutritional worth.

Exercise is just as important as a healthy diet when it comes to diabetes prevention—these two lifestyle factors go hand in hand. However, you don't need to buy new

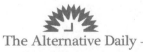

running shoes and start running marathons in order to make an active lifestyle change. In fact, a word of caution, intense training for endurance oriented events, like marathons, has a tendency to increase not just acute inflammation (all exercise basically does that) but can increase chronic inflammation in the body as well (due to extended periods of repeated acute inflammation without adequate time for the body to heal). Doing about half an hour of moderate exercise a few times a week is a great start. Walk a little more, enjoy frequent bike rides, visit your local swimming pool, or just enjoy time hiking in nature with friends and family. These activities, when performed regularly, will make a tremendous difference to your overall health.

All of the actions discussed in this chapter will not only help you lower your diabetes risk (or manage existing diabetes), they will also help you lower your risk factors for a plethora of other serious diseases. Take action, get informed, and put your health first and foremost!

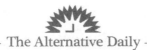

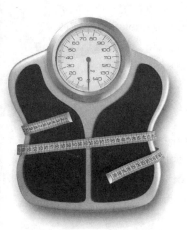

Chapter Six
Waist Not, Want Not: The Obesity Epidemic

There is no denying that obesity is a serious threat to our nation's health. Over a third of American adults are now considered obese! There are a number of reasons for these growing obesity percentages, with several underlying factors. These include poor diet, stress, certain medications and an overall sedentary lifestyle. If our nation is to become healthier, something must be done to reverse this trend.

The dieting industry makes huge profits from people wanting to lose weight, and yet, obesity rates are still on the rise. Losing weight with the help of pills, shakes or prescription drugs can be dangerous, and it's unlikely that individuals will keep the weight off. While weight loss can occur temporarily from crash diets and trends, the pounds often pile back on unless lifestyle and overall health are addressed.

To add insult to injury, the obesity crisis seems to have happened without us even realizing it. Over the last twenty years, fat-free and low-fat foods have been promoted as optimal choices for a healthy diet, yet America has become sicker, hungrier and more dependent on these packaged foods.

Starting in the 1980s, we were told by many media sources, and a number of health organizations, that less fat is better, and that cutting calories is a weight loss solution. The problem with this theory is that it does not address the quality of the calories themselves, or the fact that our bodies need calories to actually burn fat. Our bodies thrive on calories—they just need to be the right ones!

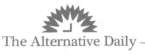

The food industry took advantage of the low-calorie trend by pumping out tons of processed options that were low in fat, yet void of nutrition. And guess what? We bought the idea. As a result, we started taking in more sugar and empty calories, and we started gaining weight. As we became more malnourished and hungrier due to these processed low-calorie foods, we also suffered a mental shift. We stopped thinking about food in terms of nutrients, and started thinking about how to consume less.

Our relationship with food has changed. After years of depriving our bodies, our metabolisms have slowed down and we have become reliant on quick sources of calories. Enter fast foods and conveniently packaged, processed meals. In essence, this is one of the major reasons America has become the fattest country in the world today.

While the processed food companies have gained from this demand for "low-fat" empty calories, the individuals eating these foods have not. People have become overweight, unhealthy, and more dependent on medical care, especially as it relates to heart disease, diabetes, high blood pressure and obesity.

The increased need for medications has led to a mentality of treating symptoms, though the underlying problem boils down to the fact that we are not giving our bodies proper sources of nutrient-dense foods. The average person spends more money on prescription drugs than they do on healthy foods. For instance, take a look at the popularity of sodas, candies, chips, cookies, packaged meals and larger-than-life, deep-fried restaurant portions.

We spend less time outdoors than ever before in history, we spend much of our days sitting around, and eat out more than we cook at home. All of these things combined have slowly but surely led us to where we are today.

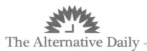

The problem of obesity demands immediate change, before our nation's health becomes even worse. While everyone knows that, no one seems to know what to do about it—or they feel as though there has been too much damage done, and there's no point in changing. Individuals suffering from obesity must make drastic lifestyle changes immediately, and these changes may seem not only daunting, but downright impossible in a system that makes it so easy to overconsume and remain underactive.

One of the most detrimental aspects of this issue is the fact that we are still often told that calories are all that matter. If it's low in calories, it must be good for us, right? This mentality is one of the main reasons that our obesity rates continue to rise. Simply looking at calories doesn't address the quality of our foods, and quality is what we need. High-quality foods—whole, nutritious, unprocessed foods—are what our bodies need to thrive.

Ultimately, two types of changes need to occur if we are to face obesity head-on. Firstly, we've got to change the way we think about food, calories and quality. Secondly, we've got to change the way we eat and the way we choose to fuel our bodies.

Syndrome X

Obesity has led to what we'll call Syndrome X: a mindset of overconsumption at the risk of our health, which ultimately leads to illness. This mindset began with Generation X, when low-quality convenience foods and more time spent inside became so popular. These habits have become mainstream, and have been adopted by younger generations ever since.

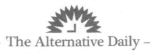

A typical restaurant meal today can contain well over 2,000 calories, many of which the body can't use as energy, and just stores as fat. Children's meals are twice the size they used to be, and are higher in empty calories too. This is not how our children should have to grow up—it is detrimental to their growth and development.

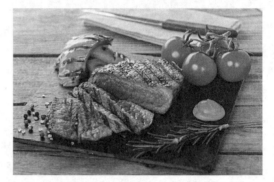

Our society's obsession with oversized portions and convenience comes at a huge cost. Most convenience foods are the least healthy options. These low-quality foods include fast food meals, sodas, chips, cookies, boxed cereals, packaged deli meals, premade pasta dishes, giant subs, tubs of deep-fried chicken and biscuits and most foods found at convenience stores. Convenience foods are largely to blame for the obesity crisis in America.

The average "9 to 5" American office worker is often affected by Syndrome X. They rush in the morning to get to the office, often grabbing a fast food breakfast, a donut, a packaged granola bar or a bowl of cereal. They load up on sugary coffee to get them through the morning, and then sit all day at their desk at work. If they even manage to get out for lunch, they're likely to grab something fast that's fried and/or high in sugar. Then they sit for the rest of the day at their desk with little activity. This routine contributes to high blood sugar, diabetes and weight gain.

As stress increases throughout the day, the average American office worker will likely turn to either more sugary coffee, or a soda, to get them through. This abundance of sugar increases the stress hormone cortisol in the body and leads to fat storage. When

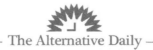

The Alternative Daily

cortisol rises and falls, it exhausts the adrenal glands, leading to an extreme onset of fatigue. This only propels the cycle even further. The exhausted worker comes home after a long day, and all they want to do is sit on the couch and eat, or go for drinks to take their mind off the stress of the day.

While this may represent a stereotype, it's a very real picture for many people. The demands of work and the stresses of modern life often cause us to make poor decisions about our health.

Stress also changes the way the beneficial bacteria in the gut function, and actually alters our entire microbiome. Our microbiome is essentially the cornerstone of good health. Fast food, convenience foods, and stress all feed harmful bacteria in the gut. Research has shown that the more good bacteria you have in your gut, the lower your weight. Good bacteria can decrease stress, burn fat and elevate your mood, leading you to make better choices. These good bacteria even counteract cravings for unhealthy foods, so you can see why they are absolutely vital for overall nutrition.

However, our diets over the last thirty years have altered the way our microbiomes work. With the nutritional decline of our diets comes the decline of the health of our microbiome. As a result, digestive problems and autoimmune disorders are on the rise, and obesity is more prevalent than ever. One of the leading causes of all these problems is also one of the hardest to overcome: our addiction to and reliance on sugar.

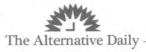

Sugar

Sugar is by far the most dangerous food we eat. It is also a leading culprit behind our expanding waistlines. Sugar triggers all the major fat-storing hormones in the body, and it leads to enhanced food cravings, fatigue and a host of body responses which lead the body to store fat.

Sugar has been found to be more addictive than cocaine, and because we can't seem to stop eating it, this legal "drug" is slowly killing us. It has been directly linked to type 2 diabetes, heart disease, binge eating, fatty liver disease, cancer and adrenal fatigue, among many other health issues.

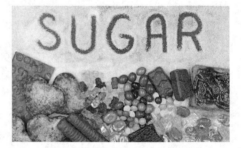

The worst part is, sugar is everywhere we look—even in some so-called healthy foods. Here are just a few of the places where sugar turns up:

- Candy bars
- Granola bars
- Granola
- Low-calorie, fiber-rich cereals
- Most cereals of any kind, organic or not
- Baked goods
- Flavored yogurts
- Sodas
- Juice

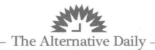

- Energy drinks

- Salad dressings

- Ketchup and barbecue sauces

- Nutrition and protein bars

- Many baking ingredients

- Frozen meals

- Frozen desserts

- Low-calorie diet foods of all kinds

- Many reduced-fat foods

- Most packaged foods

That's a long list, but it only covers some of the places you'll find sugar, because sugar is one of the sneakiest ingredients that appears on labels. It can be labeled under 57 different names, some of which sound natural, such as "evaporated cane juice," which sounds harmless enough. However, no matter what you call it, it's still sugar. Always remember that anything that contains sugar will cause your blood glucose to rise.

Let's talk for a minute about fructose. Fructose is a type of sugar found in fruits and certain vegetables (such as corn), which you'll often find in the processed form of high fructose corn syrup. Since it causes a slower rise in blood glucose levels, many people believe it's less harmful than regular sugar, but this is not the case. The body can only use so much fructose at one time, no matter how slowly it digests. Whatever the body cannot use goes straight to the liver, where it ends up being stored as fat. High fructose corn syrup has been linked to fatty liver disease, weight gain and obesity.

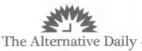

The only way you should be consuming fructose is in whole fruits and vegetables. When housed in fruits and starchy veggies, it is the most natural form of sugar, and the optimal type for humans to enjoy. Won't this form of sugar harm us, you ask? Not if you eat whole fruits and starchy veggies in moderation. Because fruits and starchy vegetables are full of fiber, vitamins and minerals, the body treats their fructose content differently.

Vegetables, including super-healthy dark leafy greens, should always be prioritized over any form of sugar, even fruit. Vegetables help to eliminate fat from the body, and also prevent sugar cravings before they start. Vegetables also help to prevent fatty liver disease, as long as you're replacing sugary foods in your diet with these optimal choices.

One of the best decisions anyone can make in order to help prevent obesity, and also to lose weight, is to start replacing all sugar-containing foods with whole, fresh vegetables. This one change would have a profound impact on both your short and long term health.

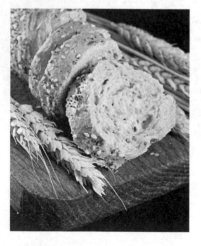

Wheat

Another important issue when it comes to weight gain is the matter of wheat and gluten. The high amount of wheat, especially refined wheat, in our diets is a contributing factor to our nation's high level of obesity.

First, the wheat we eat today is not the same wheat eaten in past generations. Because it is an easy grain to reproduce and alter to make cheap processed foods, it has become one of the most

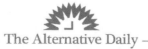

unhealthy foods in the American diet. Wheat that is highly processed is richer in gluten, a protein that has been directly linked to not only weight gain, but also to inflammation.

Next, the wheat found in the majority of processed foods (flour, cereals, cookies, chips, granola bars, etc.) triggers a huge spike in glucose levels in the body. Processed wheat products (even whole-grain breads) are quickly digested and cause a spike in blood sugar levels, at which point a significant release of insulin occurs which in turn causes the body to store fat. Any time insulin increases dramatically, fat storage will occur. Then, when insulin falls and you feel tired and hungry again, the cycle repeats itself - since you are now hungry and feel like you should eat (low blood sugar caused by spike in insulin breaking it down). Just like sugar, wheat has been found to be a highly addictive substance.

Wheat is one of the hardest foods for many people to give up because for one, it's labeled as healthy, and two, it's addictive, like most processed foods. Wheat's high gluten content also directly leads to inflammation because it is difficult for the body to process. Inflammation, in turn, often leads to weight gain. This creates the perfect setup for obesity.

Body shape

What about body shape? Are some of us more prone to weight gain than others? Perhaps, but it is not a "one size fits all" answer.

For instance, someone who has the body type known as "pear-shaped" is more prone to gain weight in the hips and thighs than in the abdominal region. This is actually one of the healthiest forms of weight gain (though possibly not ideal for many people), because fat storage in the abdominal area indicates that there is visceral (under the skin) fat directly surrounding the organs. This is a huge problem because visceral

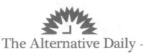

fat directly leads to health problems associated with liver disease, heart disease and diabetes, and can even hinder the reproductive organs in the body.

So, even though you may not want to gain extra pounds around your hips and thighs, it's the fat layer around your middle that you should be especially concerned about.

Individuals who tend to store fat in their abdominal region are generally referred to as "apple-shaped." While people who are apple-shaped may have to watch their weight more closely, it does not mean they were meant to be (or have to be) overweight or obese. It simply means they'll need to be more careful about their body weight, since fat storage in the abdominal region is more detrimental to a person's health.

The last type of body shape we'll talk about is the "carrot shape." These individuals are generally thin, and have little in the way of curves. Many carrot-shaped people actually have a hard time putting on weight. While they might seem lucky, this body shape is not a free pass to eat unhealthy foods. If they make unhealthy choices over time, even those with the carrot shape can become obese.

Even though excess abdominal weight is the most dangerous type, all excess body weight can contribute to health problems. As a person gains weight, their metabolism slows down, hormones change, and food cravings increase. No matter what body shape you have, controlling excess weight gain by adopting a healthy lifestyle is paramount.

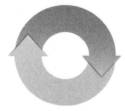

Break the cycle

Weight gain is a hard cycle to break, but making healthy choices in your daily life will keep your weight in check no matter what shape you are. The key is to choose whole, unprocessed foods and stay away from sugar and wheat. Eat a variety of

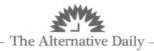

vegetables, a moderate amount of whole fruits, as well as natural, whole sources of protein and fats. Then, no matter what body shape you have, you will be caring for your body the way nature intended.

Foods that help decrease your chances of gaining weight and actually help you burn fat include the following:

- Omega-3-rich foods (walnuts, flax, chia, wild-caught fish, acai fruit)

- Leafy green vegetables

- Sweet potatoes, beets, carrots, and squash

- Whole-food sources of healthy fat (extra-virgin coconut oil, extra-virgin olive oil, grass-fed butter, and grass-fed meats and poultry)

- Gluten-free grains such as quinoa, amaranth, and steel-cut oats in place of wheat (in moderation)

- Homemade green juices (not fruit juices)

- Green smoothies

- Fermented foods (plain yogurt, kefir, kimchi and sauerkraut)

- Low-sugar fruits (berries, oranges, green apples, lemons, limes, cantaloupe, cucumber, tomato)

- Plain coffee (no sugar, please!) or coffee mixed with coconut oil

- Herbal tea

- Coconut and almond flour (in place of glutenous flours)

- Raw nuts and seeds (in moderation)

- Beans and legumes (legumes are best when sprouted)

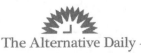

Eating the above-listed foods regularly, with a main focus on vegetables, will increase your chances of losing weight and keeping inflammatory responses to a minimum. These whole, nutritious foods will also keep you more full than processed foods, and most are very affordable. You can also prepare all of them ahead of time, as many are easy to freeze, so you're never out of options.

Remember, obesity starts with making unhealthy choices, but you can reverse the cycle by making healthy choices each day.

What kind of eater are you?

If you're reading this and wondering how your eating habits stack up, consider what type of eater you are. Are you a high-energy type who craves sugar and caffeine to get by? If so, you may benefit from more satiating—and stress relieving—meals such as overnight oats with chia and sliced fruit for breakfast, black bean salad with kale and sweet potatoes for lunch, and raw almonds for a snack. Dinner might be a nice piece of salmon, with a side of pre-made quinoa and a salad. Or leftover lentil chili—whichever you'd like.

Are you someone who does not have a high-stress job but still craves sugar and junk food? You might benefit from choosing a high-protein diet rich in healthy fats, with a lower starch and sugar content. A breakfast for you might be a smoothie containing some ground flax seeds, greens and strawberries. You could add some raw almond butter to help stabilize the hormones that lead to sugar cravings. Or, you could whip up some pastured eggs with kale, cooked in coconut oil. Lunch could be wild fish with kale and avocado, or an avocado salad with tomatoes, quinoa and cucumber. A great snack would be low in sugar and rich in protein, such as organic Greek yogurt sweetened with unprocessed stevia and cinnamon, with a side of a few walnuts and sliced

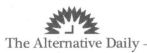

carrots. Dinner should be rich in protein and vegetables, such as black bean chili with vegetables of your choice, or maybe a wild-caught salmon steak with a side of quinoa, green beans and leafy greens.

Individuals who crave sugar should prioritize lean proteins, moderate amounts of healthy fats, and plenty of vegetables and greens in their diet. Those who simply eat junk out of lack of time or stress should try instead to eat foods that are high in protein, gluten-free complex carbs and non-starchy vegetables to reduce stress and aid in satiety.

How does this work exactly? The amino acids in protein stabilize cravings, optimize hormonal function and enhance metabolism. When the body receives proper nutrition, sugar cravings are naturally reduced. Since stress can trigger sugar cravings, it is vital to eat in a way that decreases stress and cravings at the same time.

Thinking about what type of eater you are, and getting to the root of your cravings, may help you make the necessary changes to reverse your unhealthy food habits and begin living a healthier life.

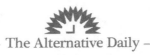

Chapter Seven
Leaky Pipes: Inflammation and Digestive Disturbances

We live in a society where to-do lists and stress levels appear to be the measurements of human productivity. Whether in regards to our personal schedule or our work schedule, if we're not fully booked and worn out, we feel like we're not making the most of our time. The increasing pace of our everyday lives can wreak havoc on our health, leading to digestive problems, depression and a series of inflammatory and autoimmune disorders.

You see, our modern world has become polluted as a result of rapid growth and the increasing demands of our everyday lives. Our bodies have become polluted as well. For corporate convenience, cost savings and business growth, our food is now genetically altered, pumped with hormones, injected with artificial colors and flavors, and covered with preservatives. Our water and air are full of toxins and allergens. On top of that, we are stressed—highly stressed.

As a result, our own cells have turned against us. Our bodies view these environmental toxins and food chemicals as dangerous intruders, and begin pumping out white blood cells and antibodies to protect us. And while our intestinal flora is full of microscopic life forms that assist our immune system in fighting harmful substances, the stress, toxins and lifestyle choices we make cause an imbalance in our gut, which then turns against us, weakening our bodies ability to fight off debilitating diseases.

No one seems to have time to relax anymore, or even to eat properly and sleep at night. Families have traded time together at the park for time around the television set. Home-cooked meals have been replaced with fast food and microwavable instant dishes. Although these luxuries make life more convenient, and therefore less emotionally stressful at times, they add more overall stress to our body. A sedentary

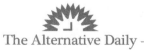

lifestyle, in which work is performed at a desk and rest involves vegetating on the couch, has become a dangerous norm. Our country's rates of obesity, degenerative diseases, and inflammatory ailments are through the roof. In the process of taking care of our futures, we have forgotten to take care of ourselves.

As we have mentioned, boxed, canned, frozen, instant, or drive-thru meals are packed with artificial ingredients, hormones, antibiotics and carcinogens. Any one of these types of additives can cause an autoimmune response, and yet they are all found in so many common, everyday meals, snacks and drinks. Researchers are finding a direct correlation between the food we eat and our ability to fend off deadly bacteria, viruses, allergens and fungi.

We are all fighting for time, however, the best way to have more time for the things that really matter is to live a more balanced, healthy life. It sounds counterintuitive, but when we rush our lives away, we have less time because we are sick more often and are more likely to die at a younger age due to poor diet, stress and a lack of exercise and rest. You can extend the amount of productive time you have by making better lifestyle choices, which in turn helps to ensure that your body can take care of you. Not only will achieving good health allow you more productive time, it will allow you more time to enjoy your life, as well!

A healthy immune system is in large part the result of a healthy gut, and a healthy gut is a direct result of your actions. Treat your gut well and it will reward you with a body that is more efficient and effective, allowing you to thrive.

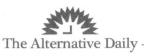

The importance of healthy gut flora (a delicate balance)

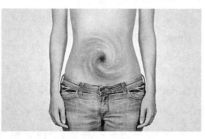

Researchers are beginning to link more and more chronic and debilitating diseases to inflammation of the gut due to an autoimmune response. Digestive disorders such as irritable bowel syndrome, food allergies, inflammatory bowel disease, Crohn's disease, candida and GERD are being diagnosed at an alarming rate. Seemingly unrelated diseases of the brain, heart, bones and nervous system are also now understood as being connected to the bacteria in our gut, and our immune system as a whole. Diseases such as heart disease, cancer, diabetes, arthritis, Alzheimer's disease, Parkinson's disease and depression have also all been linked to gut inflammation and the immune system.

A 2008 study published by the National Center for Health Statistics revealed that incidents of food allergies in children rose by 18 percent from 1997 to 2006. Diagnosed celiac disease has quadrupled over the past 50 years. Diabetes is projected to increase 165 percent by 2050, according to a study published by the American Diabetes Association.

The World Health Organization expects global cancer rates to increase 50 percent by 2020. The Endocrine Society released a paper suggesting that diabetes complications can lead to a higher risk of dementia. Not surprisingly, the World Health Organization expects global dementia cases to triple by 2050. The leading cause of death in America—and in the world—is heart disease. Deaths due to heart disease increased globally by 41 percent from 1990 to 2013. As we've discussed, all of these illnesses are associated, in some way, with inflammation.

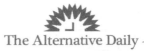

When our gut does not contain enough beneficial flora to protect it, it becomes inflamed as a result of harmful invaders, and our white blood cells begin firing. White blood cells and antibodies exist to protect our bodies from invading toxins, including bacteria, viruses and fungi. Not surprisingly, most digestive disorders have yeast, fungi or imbalanced bacteria at their root. You see, not all bacteria is bad. In fact, we need good bacteria to keep our digestive system flowing normally, to protect our immune system, and to synthesize essential vitamins such as biotin, vitamin B12 and vitamin K.

Why does gut bacteria have such an impact on the whole body? Our vital organs are all connected. Each bodily system affects the other. Our gut is like a pipe system. If toxins and harmful chemicals are not halted by our bacterial barrier, those attackers can spread through our "leaky pipes" and strike susceptible parts of our body. Since all of the above-mentioned diseases can occur as a result of our body's autoimmune responses to invaders, we need to arm our most precious inner soldier, our gut flora, with the good bacteria it needs to remain vigilant.

According to The Physicians Committee, 90 percent of our cells are microbial cells, and our diet has a direct impact on our microbes. In other words, we really are what we eat. When we eat heavily-processed, genetically-modified junk food, we damage our cells, and this may cause our immune system to turn on our own cells. The unhealthy foods we consume become the enemy, triggering inflammation and disease.

This autoimmune response can be prevented by eating natural, whole foods that nourish our bodies, provide the nutrition we need to fight off infection and disease, and keep all of our systems functioning normally. There are also foods that directly provide good bacteria to our gut, such as naturally fermented foods, which

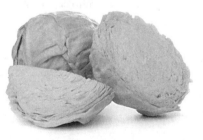

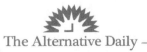

have probiotic properties. Eating prebiotic foods, such as onions, garlic, asparagus and cabbage, helps to feed beneficial bacteria, which in turn act as a shield against disease. Our intestinal flora fights against harmful intruders, ranging from influenza to carcinogens!

Our intestinal flora is very delicate, and it can easily be set off-balance. To maintain a well-balanced flora, you must live a more balanced life. Eating a more natural, nutritious diet is key, as is consuming fermented or probiotic-rich foods, and prebiotic foods. Stress, lack of sleep, and a sedentary lifestyle can also contribute to an inflamed gut. Although there are many symptoms and conditions associated with an unbalanced gut, we are going to delve deeper into the digestive disturbances that can be directly caused by a bacterial imbalance, and the autoimmune response that triggers inflammatory diseases of the gastrointestinal tract, or GI tract.

Irritable Bowel Syndrome (IBS)

Irritable bowel syndrome is a medical term that is used as a blanket explanation for a series of otherwise unexplained symptoms caused by the inflammation of the large intestine. One third of the population has experienced IBS at some point, but only one in 10 people experience severe enough symptoms to seek medical help. These symptoms can include abdominal pain or spasms that are relieved after a bowel movement, bloating, abdominal swelling, excessive gas, stomach rumbling, a feeling of urgency to use the bathroom, incontinence, sharp pain inside the rectum, a sensation of incomplete bowel movement, diarrhea, constipation and alteration of bowel habits.

Unlike other inflammatory diseases of the intestines, IBS does not damage your gut, nor does it increase your chances of developing cancer or other bowel conditions. However, symptoms do not only occur in the intestines. Sometimes symptoms can occur in other parts of the body, and may include headaches, backaches, muscle

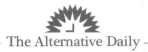

pain, joint pain, nausea, frequent urination, belching, shortness of breath, anxiety, depression, dizziness and fatigue.

This range of symptoms is also often experienced by those who have been diagnosed with fibromyalgia, functional dyspepsia, anemia, celiac disease, inflammatory bowel disease (IBD) and chronic fatigue syndrome. Researchers are discovering deeper connections between these various disorders due to chronic gut inflammation. It is therefore not surprising that symptoms may overlap with other inflammatory disorders, even those that are not directly connected to intestinal problems.

If you are experiencing any of these symptoms, it is important that you do not try to self-diagnose, as these symptoms can also be a sign of other problems. Instead, pay a visit to a qualified medical professional. According to the International Foundation for Functional Gastrointestinal Disorders, IBS is diagnosed by evaluating the symptoms, undergoing laboratory blood and stool tests, X-rays and endoscopic procedures, such as a colonoscopy. These tests can assist a gastrointestinal specialist in ruling out other diseases that present similar symptoms.

At any given time, between 10 and 20 percent of people in Western countries fulfill the criteria to be diagnosed with IBS. IBS is observed more frequently in women than in men, and is more prominent in young people than the elderly. This may be due to a combination of poor diet and stress from society's expectations.

According to the IBS Network, these two factors actually intertwine. Stress often affects the bowels, making them more sensitive and intolerant to certain foods. Also, both stress and diet alone can cause inflammation and autoimmune responses. Coffee, high-fiber foods, spices and fatty foods are often

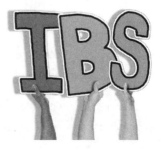

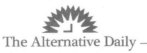

triggers for flare-ups. Instead of eliminating these foods from your diet, the IBS Network recommends adopting a more balanced diet that includes more soluble fibers from rolled oats, bananas and beans. However, if the fatty foods you are eating are processed or high in sugar, as we've discussed, it's important to stop eating them and replace them with natural sources.

Candida

Candida is a genus of yeasts. It describes over 20 yeasts that can cause infection in humans. Many candida yeasts live on the skin and mucous membranes without causing infection. However, when these yeasts become overgrown, symptoms often develop. The term "candida" as it is used most commonly is actually only one of the numerous candida yeasts known as *Candida albicans*.

Candida albicans is part of the gut flora. Overpopulation of this form of candida can weaken the intestinal wall, allowing it to infiltrate the bloodstream and release toxic byproducts throughout the body. As a result, this causes yeast overgrowth in various parts of the body, which can trigger a wide array of inflammatory symptoms. *Candida albicans* in and of itself is not necessarily a bad thing—problems arise when it grows out of control and spreads into the bloodstream.

Candida overgrowth symptoms include brain fog, feeling "drunk," sinus infections, oral thrush, persistent vaginal infections, recurring urinary tract infections, hormonal imbalance, skin and nail fungal infections, chronic fatigue and mood disorders. Even before it reaches other parts of your body, candida overgrowth can affect the gut and cause a vast amount of intestinal distress. Symptoms include constipation or diarrhea, stomach cramps, persistent flatulence, burping and bloating.

Infections caused by candida overgrowth can occur as a result of taking antibiotics, corticosteroids, cancer treatments or birth control pills, though the most common cause

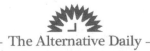

is dietary. A diet high in sugar and processed, refined, gluten-rich carbohydrates can stimulate overgrowth and infections, which in turn stimulates an inflammatory response from your weakened immune system. Individuals with autoimmune disorders and inflammatory conditions, as well as young children and the elderly, are more prone to developing a candida problem due to their weakened immune systems. People with type 1 or type 2 diabetes are also more likely to develop candida overgrowth syndrome. This is because the sugar levels in the mucous membranes of diabetics is traditionally higher than in individuals without diabetes. *Candida albicans*, like other forms of yeast overgrowth, feeds off sugar.

If you are experiencing symptoms of candida, try this at-home test—it's yucky but simple. Pour water into a glass before bedtime, and set the glass beside your bed. First thing in the morning, gather some saliva in your mouth and spit it into the glass of water. Check the glass every fifteen minutes, for a total of one hour. If you do not have candida overgrowth, the saliva should completely disappear in the water after an hour. If you have candida overgrowth, your saliva will form into one of three patterns. You may see strands of phlegm drifting downward from the top of the cup. You may also have cloudy particles suspended in the middle of the glass, or a cloud of saliva covering the bottom of the glass. Any of these suggests that you may have candida, in which case, it's time to speak with your doctor.

There are a variety of tests you may be given to confirm a candida diagnosis. Stool tests can be done to search for traces of yeast and bacteria. If your symptoms are concentrated in one area of the body, a culture may be taken to test that specific region for the presence of yeast. A blood test is ideal for wide-spread symptoms, or to see if your regional symptoms are part of a larger yeast problem. Blood may also be tested for specific antibodies. If these antibodies are abundant, then you likely have an overgrowth. Urine can also be tested for D-arabinitol, a waste product of candida. High levels of this waste product is indicative of yeast overgrowth.

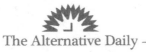

The most important change you can make when combating candida is dietary. Greatly reducing or eliminating processed, refined and gluten-rich carbohydrates is critical in preventing further growth. Also, eliminating high-glycemic foods can help further starve the yeast. Coconut oil has been found to be effective against yeast, as are foods rich in vitamin C. Supplements such as milk thistle and clove oil can also be helpful in treating candida, but speak to a health professional before trying a regimen with these. Consuming probiotic and prebiotic foods can help restore good bacteria to keep candida at bay.

Crohn's disease

Crohn's disease is a chronic disorder of the gastrointestinal (GI) tract. This disorder is named after Dr. Burrill B. Crohn, who was the first to describe the disease in 1932. Dr. Crohn and his associates also discovered that Crohn's disease belongs to a collection of conditions known as inflammatory bowel disease, or IBD.

Although Crohn's disease is most commonly found at the bottom of the small bowel known as the ileum, it can affect any part of the GI tract, from the mouth to the anus. Due to its classification as a form of IBD, Crohn's disease symptoms resemble those of other intestinal disorders, especially ulcerative colitis, or UC. This makes diagnosing Crohn's disease a challenge. There are, however, small but noticeable differences that are unique to Crohn's disease. For example, UC affects only the innermost lining of the large intestine, including the colon and rectum, whereas Crohn's may cause symptoms throughout all layers of the intestinal wall. Also, intestinal inflammation can be patchy, with some areas that are unaffected. This does not occur in patients with UC.

As many as 700,000 Americans suffer from a form of Crohn's disease. Roughly five to 20 percent of those who suffer from Crohn's disease have a direct blood relative who is also experiencing a form of inflammatory bowel disease. Risk of having the disease is

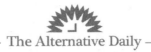

greater if both parents have a form of IBD. Genetic predisposition is more of a factor in Crohn's disease than in ulcerative colitis.

As with many diseases, genetic predisposition often needs a trigger. Stress and dietary factors can contribute to intestinal inflammation and trigger Crohn's disease or another form of IBD. These triggers also aggravate symptoms in those who have already been diagnosed. Dietary causes include eating foods that trigger inflammation or an autoimmune response, including food allergens, foods high in omega-6 fatty acids, and foods containing additives and other toxins.

Crohn's disease is found in people of all ages, but is most frequently discovered in people between the ages of 15 and 35. Crohn's disease symptoms and treatments are identical in both men and women. Symptoms mirror those of other IBD disorders, but there are also symptoms that are unique to Crohn's patients.

As mentioned before, patients with Crohn's disease may have patches of inflammation, as opposed to inflammation dispersed throughout the intestinal wall. Also, Crohn's may affect all areas of the GI tract. Symptoms unique to inflammatory diseases of the GI tract include chronic diarrhea, an urgent feeling to move bowels, abdominal cramps and pain, constipation, bowel obstruction, rectal bleeding and a sense of incomplete evacuation. Symptoms that are generally associated with IBD include weight loss, night sweats, fatigue, low energy, fever, loss of appetite and menstrual cycle irregularity.

There are five types of Crohn's disease. Understanding the symptoms and affected regions associated with each type can help patients prevent further intestinal damage, as well as alleviate symptoms. Ileocolitis is the most common form of Crohn's. It affects the region at the end of the small intestine and the start of the large intestine. Symptoms include diarrhea, cramping, pain in the right lower or middle part of the abdomen, and significant weight loss. Ileitis, another form of Crohn's disease, affects only the small intestine, but the symptoms resemble those of ileocolitis. Gastroduodenal

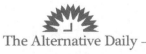

Crohn's disease affects the stomach and the upper part of the small intestine. Symptoms include nausea, vomiting, loss of appetite and weight loss. Jejunoileitis is characterized by inflammatory patches lining the upper region of the small intestine. Symptoms of jejunoileitis include mild to intense abdominal cramping and pain after meals, as well as diarrhea. Crohn's (granulomatous) colitis affects only the colon and can result in diarrhea, rectal bleeding and abscesses, and fistulas, or ulcers around the anus.

Although you can monitor your symptoms, the only way to really know if you have Crohn's disease is to see a doctor, as diagnosis often requires a series of tests. First, let your doctor know if you have a family history of inflammatory bowel disease. Next, record your symptoms over a series of two or three weeks, and note where the symptoms are occurring. Present this information to your doctor and he or she will likely run several tests.

Blood work can be helpful to test for signs of inflammation and anemia, and to rule out other conditions. Stool tests are analyzed to test for bleeding or infection due to bacteria, parasites or viruses. Barium can be delivered via an enema to allow a specialist to better view the internal organs in an X-ray. You can also have a computer tomography, or CT scan, which uses X-ray scanning and computer imaging to analyze the region. A biopsy can also be taken of the inflamed area for lab analysis. A colonoscopy is another diagnostic procedure, during which a small tube is inserted to view the rectum and intestines. There are also cameras you can ingest to record images of the digestive tract.

Foods to avoid or reduce if you have Crohn's disease include spicy foods, coffee, chocolate, carbonated beverages, alcohol, dairy and tomatoes, due to the indigestion they may cause. Also, high-fat foods such as nuts, seeds, fried foods and cured meats can cause symptom flare-ups. Edible peels from fruits and vegetables, popcorn and other foods that are harder to digest should be avoided. In contrast, almond

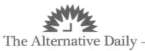

milk, eggs, rolled steel-cut oats, vegetable soups, salmon, papaya, puréed beans, poultry, avocado, butter lettuce, roasted red peppers with their skins removed, rice and nut butters are foods that are much more easily digested, and may help ease the symptoms of Crohn's disease.

Celiac and gluten sensitivity

In the case of celiac disease, an autoimmune disorder, gut bacteria stops treating gluten as food and starts treating it like an invader. As mentioned previously, gluten is a protein found in wheat, barley and rye. Gluten is found not only in these grains themselves, but also in products made from them, including white and wheat flours, pastas, bread, beer and other wheat and flour-based products. In celiac individuals, the gluten protein in these foods causes an inflammatory autoimmune response that causes the body to attack the small intestine. The effects of this are widespread and can be felt throughout the body, which makes celiac disease difficult to diagnose. Sometimes, symptoms are not felt at all.

Although there are several blood tests available to test for celiac disease antibodies, your doctor may need a biopsy of your small intestine to confirm the diagnosis. There are also labs that offer mail-in services (stool sample and genetic testing). If you have symptoms of celiac disease and yet tests are showing a negative diagnosis, you may have gluten sensitivity, also known as gluten intolerance. Gluten intolerance is the result of an autoimmune response to gluten which does not lead to intestinal damage.

Symptoms of celiac disease and gluten intolerance include chronic diarrhea or constipation, pale, fatty, or foul-smelling stool, weight loss, vomiting, irritability, fatigue, abdominal bloating, stomach pain, iron deficiency or anemia, arthritis, defects in the dental enamel of permanent teeth, canker sores in the mouth, tingling numbness in hands or feet, dermatitis herpetiformis (itchy bumps and blisters on the skin), hair loss, delayed growth and puberty, missed menstrual periods, infertility, recent miscarriage,

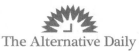

short stature, failure to thrive, bone or joint pain, bone loss or osteoporosis, seizures, migraines and attention deficit hyperactivity disorder (ADHD).

The best way to deal with a gluten problem is to eliminate gluten from your diet entirely. Unlike some of the digestive disorders mentioned in this chapter, gluten intolerance and celiac disease are chronic, lifelong conditions. A gluten-free diet ensures that the villous atrophy in the small intestine is allowed to heal, and allows symptoms to resolve themselves naturally. People with gluten 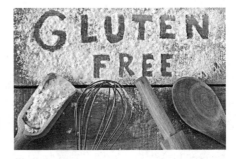 intolerance or celiac disease may also experience deficiencies in calcium, iron, zinc, folate, and vitamins B6, B12 and D.

Although these vitamin and mineral deficiencies can sometimes be rectified with a multivitamin or series of supplements, the best way to balance your gut bacteria and your entire body is to use natural, whole foods to heal from within. This way, you can have the vitamins and minerals you need (which the body absorbs better from whole foods than from supplements), plus the fiber and antioxidants of the foods in their whole form.

Processed breads, flours, pastas and specialty items must follow the Food and Drug Administration's guidelines for gluten-free processing in order for them to be labeled "gluten free." There are also a series of certifications that further protect consumers by requiring stricter guidelines than the government provides. If a product is "certified gluten-free," then you know that it exceeds or at least meets government guidelines. However, even if they're gluten-free, it is best to avoid processed products in general because of the other inflammatory additives that they may contain.

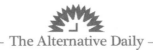

Approximately one in 100 people worldwide suffer from celiac disease. According to the *New York Times*, celiac disease has quadrupled in the United States over the last 50 years. Roughly 2.5 million Americans remain undiagnosed, and are at risk of long-term problems. You can help to prevent this disorder by reducing your consumption of processed, refined carbohydrates and gluten-rich grains, while increasing your consumption of whole foods and gut-friendly, probiotic foods.

In the final analysis, and contrary to the Food Pyramid's foundation of a significant amount of 'healthy grains' (including wheat) as part of a healthy and balanced diet - which we would firmly emphasize is very bad advice - the main glutenous culprits of wheat, barley and rye are inessential, so to be safe it is best to simply remove these from your diet. It may seem difficult at first, but with the preponderance of recent information about the downsides of gluten, coupled with public and industry acceptance resulting in a variety of alternatives, it is now much easier than it has been in the past to be gluten-free.

GERD

GERD, or gastroesophageal reflux disease, is a chronic digestive disorder that occurs when a muscle at the end of your esophagus does not close properly. This causes stomach content or acid to flow back up into your esophagus. The reflux, or backwash, irritates the lining of your esophagus and causes heartburn.

People suffering from GERD may often feel a burning sensation or pain in their chest or throat, taste stomach acid or food residue from a previous meal, experience a dry cough, have a sore throat or lump in their throat, have trouble swallowing, or experience asthma symptoms. If this happens as often as twice a week, you may be experiencing the symptoms of GERD.

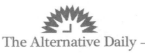

The Mayo Clinic recommends seeking medical attention specifically if you are experiencing chest pain. If chest pain is accompanied by shortness of breath, and jaw or arm pain, these are symptoms of a heart attack and not GERD. If you think you may have GERD, begin writing down symptoms, and be sure to note where you feel them in your body, the times of day that you are experiencing the symptoms, and what you ate that day. Try to recall if anyone in your family has stomach problems, as well. Your doctor may be able to diagnose GERD based on your symptoms alone.

Otherwise, your doctor may take a pH probe test to measure acid in your esophagus for 24 hours. He or she may also take an X-ray of your upper digestive tract, or take an endoscopy to visually examine inside your esophagus and stomach. A biopsy may be obtained during the endoscopy by collecting a sample of tissue for laboratory analysis. A nose catheter can also be used to measure movement and pressure in your esophagus.

There are a variety of ways to control heartburn and reduce your symptoms so that your esophagus can heal. Medications may be prescribed if the case is serious. Antacids can provide some relief, but will not heal an inflamed esophagus caused by stomach acid. If the situation is much more serious, and medication and lifestyle changes do not help, surgery to reinforce or strengthen the lower esophageal sphincter may be recommended by your specialist. To prevent further damage and truly heal your esophagus, lifestyle changes must be used in conjunction with any prescribed medications. If your situation is not serious enough for medication, dietary and lifestyle changes alone may be enough to rectify the problem.

As with other digestive problems, adapting your diet is one of the most effective ways to combat GERD. There are specific foods which can trigger acid reflux even if you are on medication for GERD. Foods to avoid include tomato sauce, garlic, onions, fatty foods, fried foods, alcohol, chocolate, mint and caffeine. You can also prevent your food from

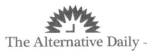

traveling up your esophagus by eating smaller meals, waiting at least three hours after eating to go to sleep, and elevating the head of your bed to prevent acid buildup while you sleep.

Maintaining a healthy weight can help you prevent your risk of many diseases, including GERD. Excess fat can put pressure on your lower abdomen, pushing your stomach and causing acid to back up into your esophagus. Smoking also prevents the lower esophageal sphincter from functioning properly, allowing acid to roam freely. Tight-fitting clothing can also put pressure on your abdomen and lower esophagus.

Along with a healthy diet, herbal remedies may be used to reduce the symptoms of GERD. These remedies include chamomile, licorice, slippery elm and marshmallow— but be sure to talk to a health professional you trust before using these, to determine which ones, and how much, is right for you. Reducing stress can also help reduce symptoms.

New research suggests that the majority of people who are diagnosed with GERD in Western society actually have NERD, or non-erosive reflux disease. This is because 70 percent of people diagnosed with GERD have no visible tissue damage, which means that their GERD symptoms are not a result of stomach acid. Instead, these individuals have a form of autoimmune disease and should not take acid-stopping drugs, because they promote bacterial overgrowth, weaken the immune system and increase symptoms. These drugs may also increase the likelihood of developing a digestive disorder, prevent the absorption of vital nutrients and increase the odds of developing cancer.

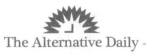

NERD symptoms mirror those of GERD, but are caused by inflammation instead of acid. Eliminating foods that trigger inflammation including allergens (such as dairy, soy and gluten), processed and refined carbohydrates and sugars, foods high in trans fats and saturated fats, omega-6 fatty acids, alcohol and monosodium glutamate (MSG) can help a lot. Foods that fight inflammation include green leafy vegetables, tea, garlic, walnuts, salmon, cherries and berries and spices like clove, ginger and turmeric.

Your risk of having GERD is increased if you are obese, pregnant, a smoker, diabetic or have scleroderma or a hiatal hernia. GERD can occur at any age, and is believed to affect 10 to 20 million Americans. Although 30 to 40 percent of acid reflux may be hereditary, food and lifestyle choices are often the cause of GERD. Regardless of your risk factors, adopting a healthy lifestyle can help prevent GERD, or manage its symptoms if you have it.

What you can do right now to tame the inflammation in your gut

If you have symptoms of a specific digestive disorder or inflammatory disease, avoiding trigger foods is key. These vary depending on what disorder you have. For instance, people suffering from GERD, Crohn's, or IBS should avoid high-fat foods, oily and fried foods, certain spices, and anything highly acidic. On the other hand, people with celiac disease, diabetes, or candida should avoid gluten and replace breads, pastas, refined flours and processed sugars with whole-food, natural sources of low-glycemic, fiber-rich carbohydrates.

It is also important to determine if your inflammation or autoimmune response is due to a food allergy (to be discussed in more detail later in this book). There are tests you can take for specific food allergens, but if you have a mild intolerance, then it might not show up in tests. Try eliminating a suspected allergen from your diet for two weeks, and then reintroduce it. Write down the changes you notice in your body, if any. If you notice that your symptoms decline or are gone when you eliminate the allergen, then your

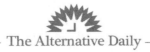

body is likely telling you that it works best when that food is eliminated from your diet. Food is fuel and nourishment for your body. Listen to your body.

As we've mentioned, some foods are inflammatory by their very nature, and should be avoided. The more refined and modified your foods are, the more likely they are to cause an autoimmune reaction. Whole foods are like a complete symphony of vitamins, minerals, enzymes, fiber, and antioxidants. When foods are processed, fortified or reconstituted, a lot of their benefits are lost. Whole foods also provide complete nutrition better than supplements or multivitamins. Your gut will thank you if you make the switch to natural, simple foods that are easy to digest and assimilate.

There are many foods that specifically work to help you combat inflammation. Just a few examples are bananas, broccoli, and cauliflower. Bananas also help stabilize gut bacteria, as do Jerusalem artichokes, which are high in fiber and powerful prebiotics. Blueberries can help boost your immune system, while cruciferous vegetables (such as kale, cabbage, Brussels sprouts, broccoli, and cauliflower) can combat the inflammatory effects of a weak immune system. Other inflammation-preventing foods include olive oil, coconut oil, amaranth, oats, leafy greens, fennel, snap peas, beets, tomatoes, nuts, wild-caught fatty fish, and fresh fruits. The natural antioxidants and polyphenols found in these foods help protect your body from chronic disease by reducing your risk of inflammation.

Prebiotic foods are simple, easy-to-digest foods that will also help balance your gut bacteria and promote a stable immune system. Prebiotics provide the building blocks for probiotics, and are easily assimilated into the body. Unlike probiotic supplements or enriched, fortified foods, prebiotic foods are rich in natural dietary fibers. These fibers include inulin, fructo-oligosaccharides, and galacto-oligosaccharides.

Vegetables that are high in these digestion-promoting fibers include Jerusalem artichokes, garlic, spring onion, fennel, chicory, leeks, shallots, cabbage, asparagus,

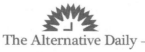

green and snow peas, and sweet corn. Prebiotic fruits include custard apples, white peaches, pomegranates, grapefruit, watermelon, rambutan, tamarillo, persimmons, and nectarines. Beans are excellent sources of prebiotic fiber, as well. Chickpeas and lentils also have prebiotic qualities. Oats, cashews, pistachios, and human breast milk are other sources of prebiotics.

Probiotic foods are foods that already have good bacteria established within their makeup. These foods are often cultured or fermented, and include fermented polenta, kimchi, sauerkraut, tempeh, natto, yogurt, coconut yogurt, kombucha tea, kvass made from beets instead of glutenous grains, kefir, coconut kefir, microalgae, dark chocolate, pickled fruits and vegetables, fermented hard-boiled eggs, and pickled fish. When it comes to these foods, however, make sure you choose whole-food varieties that have been fermented using natural methods, not processed imposters.

All in all, gut inflammation can be tamed if you pursue a balanced, natural diet and lifestyle. Slow things down, get plenty of rest at night, exercise often, and eat foods that will love you in return. Natural, whole foods, especially those high in prebiotic fiber and probiotic enzymes, can help you combat inflammation and boost your immune system. Your body may be your temple, but your gut is your shield. If you take care of it, it will take care of you.

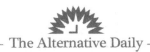

Chapter Eight
Fibromyalgia: The Mystery Condition

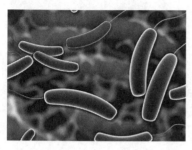

From a historical standpoint, part of the problem in diagnosing fibromyalgia has been that it is not a visible disease. The effects are obvious only to the people suffering from them. Most people with fibromyalgia appear to be well when given a physical examination. Because it is invisible to other people, it was long mistaken to be a psychosomatic condition.

Research has proven through the use of functional magnetic resonance imaging (fMRI) that people with fibromyalgia have a heightened sensitivity to pain compared to healthy people.

This is one reason why some health experts believe fibromyalgia is actually a neurosensory disorder. They believe that the central nervous system of people with fibromyalgia is interrupted or inhibited in its ability to process stimuli that indicate pain.

Research seems to indicate that the likely dysfunction results from neurochemical imbalances that amplify pain signals in the brain from one of two different inputs. The first is an increased sensitivity to stimuli that are not normally considered painful, known as allodynia. The other is hyperalgesia, a heightened response to stimuli that are painful.

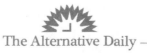

Signs and symptoms

Although symptoms may vary between individuals, the following are a few common symptoms of fibromyalgia:

- Muscle pain, stiffness or tightness
- Muscle cramps not caused by excessive exercise
- Excessive muscle and joint pain after exercise (beyond the normal "burn" that comes after a workout)
- Feeling like your hands and feet are swollen, even though they aren't
- Pain in the face and jaw
- Numbness in appendages, or in the face
- Frequent headaches or migraines
- Oversensitivity to bright light, noise or other stimuli
- Digestive disturbances
- Problems with memory
- Frequent urination
- Fatigue

These symptoms individually may indicate something other than fibromyalgia; however, if you find that you are regularly experiencing a number of them, fibromyalgia may be the culprit.

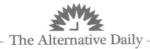

Causes

While there is no clear, definitively known cause for fibromyalgia at this time, many experts believe that sex hormones may play an important role. Fibromyalgia most commonly affects women during their middle-age years, when their sex hormones are fluctuating and beginning to decline. On top of that, a fluctuation in endocrine hormone levels due to endocrine dysfunction frequently causes similar symptoms to those found in fibromyalgia patients.

There have been indications that supplementing dehydroepiandrosterone (DHEA) may be beneficial, because of a contributing role that is believed to be played by the hypothalamic-pituitary-adrenal (HPA) axis. Stress has been associated with disruptions in the corticotropin-releasing hormone (CRH) that has direct impacts on the neuroendocrine axis.

Research has also shown that many patients with severe fibromyalgia also suffer from a growth hormone (GH) deficiency. There have been links shown between GH deficiency and elevated levels of pain severity and blood cytokines. In some studies, GH replacement therapy did appear to be linked with significant improvements to quality of life and symptoms in fibromyalgia patients with GH deficiency.

Fibromyalgia patients often have lower levels of neurotransmitters compared to healthy people. These neurotransmitters, such as norepinephrine, dopamine and serotonin, play a role in mood alterations, sleep disruptions and sensitivity to pain. These lower-than-average neurotransmitter levels imply a connection between peripheral nerve communication to the brain and fibromyalgia symptoms.

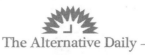

INFLAMMATION ERASED:

NATURALLY FIGHT & REVERSE DAMAGING INFLAMMATORY EFFECTS IN YOUR BODY

Fibromyalgia and inflammation

So, what's the connection between fibromyalgia and inflammation? There has been some debate on this issue throughout the years, and for a while, fibromyalgia was not considered by many health experts to be an "inflammatory condition." However, a body of recent research suggests that inflammation may indeed play an important role in both triggering and worsening this illness.

A 2012 study published in the *Journal of Neuroimmunology* analyzed the presence of certain "pro-inflammatory substances" within the spinal cord. Through this study, the researchers discovered "evidence of central inflammation" in fibromyalgia.

Another study, published in 2013 in the journal *Antioxidant & Redox Signaling,* set out to investigate "the possible relationship between mitochondrial dysfunction, oxidative stress, and inflammation in fibromyalgia." The researchers performed their study on 30 women who had been diagnosed with fibromyalgia, and used 20 women who were in good health as a control group.

On their results, the researchers wrote:

"Results lead to the hypothesis that inflammation could be a mitochondrial dysfunction-dependent event implicated in the pathophysiology of FM [fibromyalgia] in several patients indicating at mitochondria as a possible new therapeutic target."

Other studies have also indicated the presence of pro-inflammatory substances (such as cytokines, interleukin-6, and interleukin-8) in fibromyalgia patients. Research has also discovered that fibromyalgia can accompany other chronic illnesses with inflammation at their core, including arthritis and lupus. It has also been hypothesized that anti-inflammatory foods and herbs may help to mitigate fibromyalgia symptoms in some individuals.

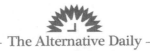

Gluten

As inflammation does indeed appear to be a prime player in fibromyalgia, avoiding glutenous grains and products becomes key in mitigating this condition. Earlier in this book, we discussed how gluten, a protein found in wheat, barley, and rye—and many processed foods—may be an inherently inflammatory substance.

For individuals who suffer from celiac disease, gluten is an utter no-no. However, even if you do not have celiac disease, gluten can be a problem. It is estimated that between 30 to 40 percent of individuals worldwide may have some degree of gluten sensitivity.

The authors of a 2014 study published in the journal *Rheumatology International* wrote:

"Fibromyalgia (FM) syndrome is a disabling clinical condition of unknown cause, and only symptomatic treatment with limited benefit is available. Gluten sensitivity that does not fulfill the diagnostic criteria for celiac disease (CD) is increasingly recognized as a frequent and treatable condition with a wide spectrum of manifestations that overlap with the manifestations of FM, including chronic musculoskeletal pain, asthenia, and irritable bowel syndrome."

To test the effects of gluten on fibromyalgia patients, the researchers involved in the study recruited 20 individuals diagnosed with fibromyalgia—none of whom suffered from celiac disease—and placed them on a gluten-free diet. The researchers followed up with the individuals for an average of 16 months, and found that many of them showed significant improvements, such as lessened pain and the ability to return to work. Some also stopped their use of opioid painkillers.

Based on their results, the study authors wrote:

"This observation supports the hypothesis that non-celiac gluten sensitivity may be an underlying cause of FM [fibromyalgia] syndrome."

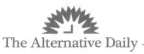

As we briefly went over earlier in this book, wheat can lead to an inflammatory response in the body in a number of ways. The gliadin portion of the gluten protein has been found to potentially permeate the intestinal barrier. This allows wheat lectins to enter the bloodstream, which can trigger inflammation.

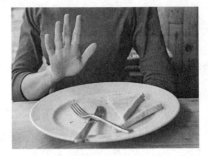

Aside from the gluten content, it is important to note that wheat can be inflammatory in other ways, as well. Wheat contains a complex carbohydrate known as amylopectin A, which causes blood sugar to spike when it is consumed, in a similar fashion as eating sugar. These rapid blood sugar spikes may trigger inflammation in the body, which if left unmitigated, may lead to chronic inflammatory illnesses, as well as insulin resistance, belly fat and digestive disturbances.

Reduce symptoms naturally

If you have been diagnosed with fibromyalgia or are experiencing fibromyalgia symptoms, the first important step you can take is to gear your lifestyle towards stopping inflammation at its source. The following are just a few things you can do:

⬥ Avoid processed foods, including refined oils.

⬥ Eat a healthy diet of anti-inflammatory foods, including plenty of fresh fruits, vegetables and sprouted legumes, along with healthy proteins and natural, unprocessed fats. Also be sure to include foods high in anti-inflammatory omega-3 fatty acids, such as wild-caught salmon, flax seeds and chia seeds.

⬥ Add plenty of anti-inflammatory herbs and spices to your meals, such as turmeric, cayenne pepper, cinnamon, clove, ginger and oregano.

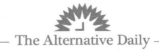

- Drink at least eight glasses of filtered water each day.

- Be sure to get at least 20 minutes of moderate exercise each day (check with your health professional of choice for options which align with your health status), as lack of physical activity is implicated in fibromyalgia.

- Ensure that you are getting between seven and eight hours of restful sleep each night.

- Make a plan to actively manage your stress. Yoga, meditation and t'ai chi are a few great, time-tested options.

We know that some of these suggestions have already been mentioned earlier—however, it's worth the repetition, as they are so crucially important for both managing fibromyalgia symptoms and for your optimal health.

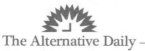

Chapter Nine
Can't Touch This: Food Intolerances and Allergies

Do you have a food intolerance or allergy? If you do, you are not alone. If you don't think you have a food allergy or intolerance, it is possible that you do and do not realize it. Food allergies and intolerances have become the topic of much discussion and research lately, because the serious health effects they may cause can be life-changing.

The term "food allergy" is defined by the National Institute of Allergy and Infectious Diseases as "an adverse health effect arising from a specific immune response that occurs reproducibly on exposure to a given food." If you have a food allergy or intolerance, or think that you might, it should be cause for concern. According to the CDC, allergies are the sixth most common cause of chronic illness in the United States.

You may have friends or family members with a food allergy or intolerance, and many people consider this a minor problem. However, the serious nature of the health risks involved is nothing to laugh at. The CDC compiled statistics on food allergies and intolerances and found that "more than 50 million Americans suffer from allergies each year." The high percentage of food allergy and intolerance cases discovered each year is staggering, and the economic cost is just as high as the health cost. The United States spends well over 18 billion dollars per year on the chronic illnesses associated with food allergies and intolerances.

Staying away from the food or foods in question is often the only way to manage symptoms. Many people find that they have these allergies during childhood, and learn to naturally stay away from "trigger" foods. However, sometimes, allergies and intolerances are not discovered until later in life, because symptoms may be mistaken for another condition.

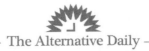

The symptoms of a food allergy range from mild to severe, depending on the person. Most food allergies trigger the immune system, and involve an immediate inflammatory response by the body. Food intolerances, on the other hand, do not involve the immune system, and instead elicit a toxic response - which are typically much more difficult to discover. As a result, food intolerances may cause more serious long-term health problems than food allergies because they are hidden or don't seem as serious.

Food intolerances, along with causing physical health issues, can also affect your psychological well-being. A 2009 study published in *Deutsches Ärzteblatt International* found that "chronic physical distress such as a food intolerance is in itself also a psychological stressor which compromises quality of life and can secondarily induce or exacerbate depression and anxiety disorders." Food intolerances are an all-around mental and physical health issue.

When your body becomes inflamed after ingesting a food allergen, you become susceptible to all of the other repercussions of inflammation, as well. These include, as we've discussed, a higher risk of chronic illness and compromised digestive function. A 2015 study published in *Gastroenterology* states, "The immediate allergic reaction leads to intense inflammation that can become life-threatening. The release of vasoactive mediators into the circulation can lead to vascular collapse and anaphylactic shock." If not addressed quickly by medical professionals, these reactions can be fatal.

Food allergies and your immune system

While your immune system operates throughout your entire body, recent research has found that approximately 70 percent of your immune function takes place in your gastrointestinal system. Given this statistic, it is no wonder why the foods we eat have such an impact on our body's defenses.

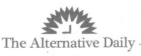

A 2008 study published in *Clinical & Experimental Immunology: The Journal of Translational Immunology* states, "The gastrointestinal system plays a central role in immune system homeostasis. It is the main route of contact with the external environment and is overloaded every day with external stimuli, sometimes dangerous as pathogens (bacteria, protozoa, fungi, viruses) or toxic substances, in other cases very useful as food or commensal flora."

The correlation between your immune system and gastrointestinal system can be seen clearly when a food allergen is consumed. Like a bullet train, the food allergen speeds to the gastrointestinal tract, triggering inflammation. The inflammation caused by food allergens often happens 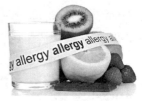 within seconds of contact between the allergen molecules and your body.

Food allergy symptoms and effects

Food allergy symptoms vary greatly. However, there are a few common symptoms that you should be on the lookout for, such as an upset stomach, vomiting, diarrhea, hives, rashes and trouble breathing. The time it takes for an allergen to affect someone varies, depending on the severity of each individual case. There are three main factors involved in the rate and severity of an allergic response: age, the allergen in question, and the amount consumed.

Even if you don't have any signs or history of food allergies, you may still be at risk. Food allergies and intolerances can occur at any age, and some are minor enough that you may not notice the symptoms. On this subject, research from Johns Hopkins Medicine found that "first-time occurrence can happen at any age, or recur after many years of remission. Allergies tend to run in families. Hormones, stress, smoke, perfume, or environmental irritants may also play a role in the development or severity of allergies."

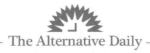

Foods that may cause allergies

There are over 140 foods that have been associated with allergic reactions—which may make singling out the cause of your food allergy or intolerance seem somewhat daunting. However, the CDC has found eight specific foods to be the cause of approximately 90 percent of all food allergy responses:

- Cow's milk

- Hen's eggs

- Peanuts

- Fish

- Wheat

- Shellfish (i.e., shrimp, prawns, crab and lobster)

- Nuts (i.e., hazelnuts, walnuts, pecans, almonds, cashews and pistachios)

- Soy products

While some of the above-listed foods are perfectly healthy for people who are not allergic to them (especially organic milk, free-range eggs, wild-caught fish and nuts), they may be quite dangerous to those that are. It's important to listen to your body carefully. If you don't feel good after eating a certain food—even if the reaction is not extreme—try cutting it out of your diet and note if you feel better.

Another key factor in food allergies is how the food is processed, packaged, prepared, stored and handled. Food reacts differently to specific manufacturing processes, and some may change their molecular structure, thus giving them a higher potential for a food allergy response.

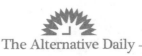

Food intolerances

A food intolerance is a toxic response by the body to a specific food or food additive. Rather than triggering the immune system, food intolerances are associated with the digestive system, as they inhibit your body's ability to digest certain foods properly. For proper digestive function, you need a balanced amount of enzymes. When enzymes become too low in number to break down the food in your gut, your digestion can go awry. Food intolerances wreak havoc on these essential enzymes needed for healthy digestion.

The American Academy of Allergy, Asthma and Immunology states, "A food intolerance, or a food sensitivity, occurs when a person has difficulty digesting a particular food. This can lead to symptoms such as intestinal gas, abdominal pain or diarrhea." While these are the common, mild symptoms of a food intolerance, symptoms may be more severe in some cases.

The following are the four most common food intolerances that affect Americans:

Lactose. Lactose intolerance affects nearly 10 percent of all adults. The response to lactose in sensitive individuals often includes diarrhea, gas, and bloating. If you are sensitive to lactose, you'll want to steer clear of cow's milk, and foods that contain it.

Tyramine. Tyramine is a component of the amino acid, tyrosine. Individuals who are sensitive to this compound may have symptoms of hives, migraines, swelling, and/or asthma. Foods that contain tyramine include fermented cheese, chocolate, red wine, sour cream, beer, yeast and avocados.

Preservatives and additives. Food intolerances to certain preservatives and additives are very common, especially since so much of today's food is loaded with unpronounceable chemicals. Benzoates, sulfites, flavoring agents like salicylates, and

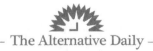

food dyes are just a few common allergens that processed foods contain. It is essential to read product labels so that you know what you are putting into your body. Avoiding processed food entirely is the best way to steer clear of potentially allergenic additives.

Gluten. Gluten intolerance has become a topic of much discussion in recent years, and has been the subject of a significant amount of research. According to the Academy of Nutrition and Dietetics, over 18 million Americans are intolerant of gluten. As we mentioned earlier, gluten is everywhere, including many foods, medications, vitamins, and even beauty products. Foods containing gluten include wheat, rye, barley, wheat germ, bulgur, farina, graham flour and a wide array of processed foods (containing any of these).

On the subject of wheat, our country's main source of gluten, the authors of a 2013 study published in *Nutrients* wrote:

"The consumption of wheat, but also other cereal grains, can contribute to the manifestation of chronic inflammation and autoimmune diseases by increasing intestinal permeability and initiating a pro-inflammatory immune response."

Food Allergies and Inflammation

As we've discussed, food allergies directly affect your immune system and often elicit inflammatory reactions. Inflammation in specific areas of the body may cause different symptoms, some minor and some severe.

These are the symptoms to look out for if you suspect a certain food allergy or intolerance:

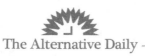

Joint inflammation. Joint inflammation is characterized by pain, stiffness or swelling in the joints. It may also develop into arthritis over time if it is not addressed.

Skin inflammation. Skin inflammation is a common telltale sign of a food allergy. Some common manifestations include hives, eczema and psoriasis.

Brain membrane inflammation. This type of inflammation may lead you to experience headaches, and in more serious cases, migraines.

Lung inflammation. A person experiencing a food allergy response in the lungs may have trouble breathing as their heart rate increases, making lung inflammation especially dangerous. This type of inflammation may also cause respiratory congestion, a chronic cough, and even asthma.

Nervous system inflammation. Inflammation in the nervous system is also very dangerous. If left unchecked, this type of inflammation may lead to serious conditions such as multiple sclerosis and epilepsy.

Some food allergies and intolerances are obvious, while others are not. If you think you may be allergic to a certain food, but aren't sure, there are a few things you can do. A medical professional can run tests for some allergens, but if the allergy is minor, it may not show up. At home, you can try eliminating a certain food from your diet for two weeks, and then reintroducing it into your diet. Take note of how you feel during the break from the food, and when you start eating the food again.

If you find that you feel better when a certain food is not on your plate, your body may well be telling you to stay away from it. Avoiding a food you are allergic or intolerant to—even if the symptoms are minor—may help you reduce your risk of a number of chronic illnesses.

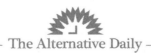

Steps you can take

If you are not sure what foods may be causing you to have food allergy symptoms, talk to your doctor about getting some allergy tests done. The IgG allergy blood test reads your IgG antibody response to a wide variety of foods. This food allergy test can help you to narrow down the foods that you need to start eliminating from your diet.

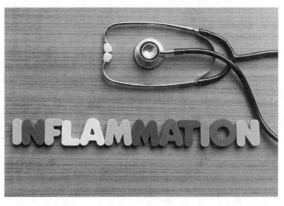

Putting your diet first and foremost will allow you to begin your fight against food allergy symptoms and inflammation. Obviously, once you know which foods are causing the problem, it is important to avoid them.

Also, enliven your diet with plenty of vegetables, fruits, healthy proteins, and whole, nutritious fats. Making sure you eat a bounty of fruits and vegetables can help you fight inflammation, as they contain a wealth of anti-inflammatory antioxidants. Avoid trigger foods and processed junk, and make your diet as varied, exciting, and healthy as you can!

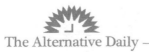

Chapter Ten
Cancer: Cells Gone Wild

*I*nflammation and cancer both significantly disturb the balance and health of an organism. So, what's the connection? Research shows that the two may be more connected than you think.

Ayurvedic medical practitioners 5,000 years ago understood the concept that prolonged cellular irritation can lead to cancer. About 2,000 years ago, a Greek physician named Claudius Galenus reported on the similarities he observed between cancerous tissues and inflamed tissues.

In the 1860s, a German scientist named Rudolf Virchow also suggested a link, detailing his observations of white blood cells, known as leukocytes, at the site of tumors. He also observed that cancer developed at the same sites where chronic inflammatory conditions were found. The link between cancer and inflammation is now being examined in more detail by modern researchers.

Cancer on the rise

Research on the prevention and treatment of cancer has intensified, as cancer rates are increasing dramatically worldwide, and especially across developed nations. The World Health Organization (WHO) 2014 World Cancer Report predicted that cancer rates would rise 57 percent over the next 20 years. In 2012, there were approximately 14 million cancer cases, with 8.2 million deaths. By 2032, these figures are expected to rise to 22 million cases, with 13 million deaths annually.

The number of newly diagnosed cancer cases is increasing, but fortunately, survival rates are also increasing. The rate of life expectancy is on the rise and has climbed steadily over the past few generations.

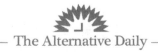

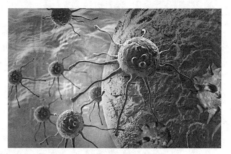

Populations around the world are growing and aging, so these figures are not altogether surprising. However, there is still such an immense number of people with cancer needing treatment, which puts a great amount of pressure on economies. Cancer was estimated to cost 1.16 trillion dollars in 2010. Christopher Wild, director of the International Agency for Research on Cancer, stated that a renewed focus on prevention will be necessary since "we cannot treat our way out of the cancer problem."

Public health initiatives in places like the United States have lessened exposure to tobacco smoke—a contributing factor to cancer—by banning public smoking in some areas and increasing taxes on tobacco products. The WHO has indicated that the next step will be to implement similar measures for toxic substances such as sugary drinks, occupational and environmental carcinogens, and air pollution.

The World Cancer Report indicated that the heaviest burden will be placed on developing countries, where there are the least resources to deal with increasing cancer rates. These nations have populations that are living longer, but at the same time becoming more vulnerable to cancers stemming from factors related to industrialized lifestyles.

As cancer continues to be a human health crisis worldwide, the link between cancer and inflammation has become a hot research topic. Let's dive a little deeper into this topic.

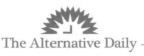

Cancer cells recruit the body's inflammatory process for their own use

As we've discussed, the body's innate process of inflammation, in the short term, serves to protect us from illness, fights off invading pathogens, and helps to heal damaged tissues. Acute inflammation in the body is perfectly healthy and necessary for survival.

In fact, a recent study by neuroscientists at the Lerner Research Institute at the Cleveland Clinic in Ohio found that allowing the acute inflammatory process to run its course actually promotes better and faster healing. One of the leading researchers explained that any treatment should be applied carefully, so that the body's own inflammatory mechanisms can still exert their benefit.

While this immune process is very effective for the healing of damaged tissues, it unfortunately seems that cancerous cells are able to hijack the system for their own benefit. Current theories indicate that after a tumor has reached a certain size, it can no longer collect the oxygen and nutrients it needs from its immediate environment. When this happens, the tumor starts to build an infrastructure for itself by recruiting the body's processes and turning them to "the dark side."

Cancer cells send out chemical signals to attract immune cells called macrophages and granulocytes to the tumor area. When these signals are sent out, immune cells cells react the same way they do when they are called to the site of an injury or illness, as explained above. They start the growth of new blood vessels to heal the area in a process called angiogenesis. Originally, this was seen by the scientific community as an effort by the immune system to attack the tumor and regenerate the tissue. However, it is now understood that the new blood vessels actually bring in oxygen and nutrients which the tumor then uses for growth.

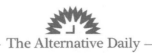

This process is the beginning of the recruitment of the body's own inflammatory response and immune system to increase the growth of cancer. There are at least six other mechanisms used in this process:

The stroma: Immune cells secrete molecules called cytokines, which inflame the tissue surrounding the injury site (in this case, the tumor). This forms a cushion called the stroma, which would normally protect an area requiring healing. However, in this case, the tumor uses it as structural support.

Oncogenes: A microenvironment of chronic inflammation turns on oncogenes, which are genes that turn cells into tumors.

Free radicals: Some of the body's inflammatory cells try to attack the tumor with weapon molecules called free radicals, but these just serve to damage the surrounding tissue and make it ripe for the growth of cancer.

Metastasis: The latest theories indicate that the inflammatory process is also the key to the way that cancer spreads throughout the body. When tumor cells are able to leave the original site and establish growth in additional areas, this is called metastasis. It is believed that some chemicals produced in the inflammatory process help the tumor cells physically cut loose from their surroundings by removing molecular "tethers."

Resistance to anti-growth and cell death signals: In a healthy situation, any abnormal or damaged cells are controlled via sophisticated signalling, which tells those cells to stop growing and even to die. They are then swept away in the body's natural clean-up processes. Cancerous growths are able to resist these signals, resulting in a large number of cells which have escaped the normal growth control mechanisms.

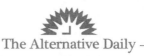

Escaping surveillance: Since a tumor involves the body's own cells, it is able to "fly under the radar" and avoid being sensed as a foreign entity. In this way, it avoids being attacked by the immune system.

How cancer spreads

Cancer originates at one site in the body, where cells have begun to mutate and malfunction. This is called the primary cancer, or primary site. As mentioned above, inflammatory and immune processes may help cancerous cells to break off from this original location and spread through the body. If this happens, 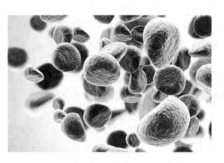 the additional sites are called metastases. The process undergone by the cancer in order to travel to different sites is called metastasis.

In a normal situation, cells are held in place by a structure called the basement membrane. Tumor cells grow through this membrane using the subversive mechanisms described above. If some cells are able to break off from the original tumor, they can travel through either the blood circulatory system or the lymph system, and start to grow additional tumors.

Cancer cells which move around via the blood are called circulating tumor cells. Research is currently searching for a way to locate these circulating cells to avoid more invasive tests such as biopsies, and to determine the best treatment method for each individual patient.

A circulating cell finishes its journey when it gets stuck in a small capillary. It must then migrate through the blood vessels to the tissue of a nearby organ, where it may be

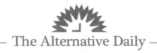

able to establish itself for further growth. Most tumor cells do not survive this process, and are either killed by white blood cells or physically destroyed by the journey. They do, however, have one sneaky trick which helps them find new host tissue. Circulating tumor cells can sometimes attach to platelets, which are cells that help blood to clot. These are eventually filtered out by capillary networks, so tumor cells may hitch a ride into surrounding tissues right along with them.

The second way that cancer cells may spread is through the lymphatic fluid. The body's lymphatic system is a network of tubes joined by lymph nodes and glands that serve to filter fluids and fight infection. Lymph fluid is a carrier medium for damaged or harmful cells that need to be removed. Cancer cells are usually part of this dangerous cargo to be shipped out. However, these cells occasionally become trapped inside of a lymph gland and cannot be destroyed. Instead, they are able to establish additional growth sites (metastases).

A third type of spread is called micrometastases. This is where tiny cancer cells float throughout the body's fluid systems, but cannot be detected on a scan. Sometimes doctors are able to perform blood tests which can read proteins given off by cancer cells, which indicate that micrometastases are present. Usually, however, the presence of micrometastases can only be predicted on the basis of a number of other factors, such as the grade of abnormality in the cancer cells, and whether any cancerous cells were found in blood vessels or lymph pathways when a previous tumor was removed. Often, precautionary medical treatment is prescribed if micrometastases are suspected, since these tiny cells may be in the process of spreading cancer somewhere in the body.

Metastatic spread is often responsible for the return of cancers after they are thought to have been eradicated.

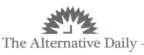

Link between chronic inflammatory conditions and cancer

A 2015 study published by researchers at MIT pinpointed the link between chronic inflammatory diseases and the development of cancer. For example, diseases like colitis, pancreatitis and hepatitis have been linked with a greater risk for cancers of the colon, pancreas and liver. This is because these inflammatory conditions may set the scene for genetic mutations which are part of the cancer process.

These inflammatory conditions may do this by causing immune cell activity, which in turn may lead to cell division and the production of reactive molecules that can damage DNA. Cells which are in the process of dividing are more vulnerable to DNA damage, and therefore to mutations that can lead to cancer. The MIT researchers used a new type of technology to display this pathway—they were able to use a biologically engineered mouse with fluorescing genes to control the onset of inflammation, and then read DNA damage markers and mutations in tissue.

The researchers then experimented with the correlation between timing of inflammation and number of mutations. They found that there is a delay between the onset of inflammation and the beginning of cell division—a protective mechanism for those sensitive dividing cells. However, when another round of inflammation happens too soon after this process, the cells that are in the middle of division may get caught in the inflammatory conditions, and are more prone to mutation.

The MIT team found that chronic or repeated inflammatory episodes (such as those seen in colitis, pancreatitis, hepatitis or other inflammatory conditions such as arthritis and psoriasis) led to a significant increase in damaging mutations because of the way that sensitive cells, which should be busy repairing tissues post-inflammation, are left vulnerable by the next oncoming inflammatory episode.

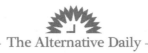

This correlation was found in mice, but the MIT researchers indicated that the effect could potentially be even more pronounced in humans, because of the way that modern life often predisposes us to chronic or repeated inflammation for years or decades at a time.

Research published in the journal *Oncology* supports the idea that the longer an inflammatory condition persists, the greater the risk of associated cancerous changes at the cellular level. Crohn's disease and ulcerative colitis have been studied in particular, as precursors of colorectal cancer. Research suggests that people with these inflammatory conditions have five to seven times the risk of developing cancer after having the condition for at least eight years. It has been observed that cancerous cells tend to appear at the site of the chronic inflammation (in a process called neoplasia) after an average of 15 years if Crohn's or colitis is left unchecked.

Chemical exposure on top of inflammation increases risk of cancer

The same MIT study mentioned above found that exposure to DNA-damaging chemicals from the external environment serves as a "double whammy" for those who are dealing with inflammation. Many chemicals present in the environment may increase the chance of the mutations which lead to cancer.

Specifically, the researchers studied the effects of exposure to a type of chemical called an alkylating agent, which causes damage to DNA. This type of chemical is found in some foods, cosmetics, environmental toxins and pharmaceuticals.

Healthy tissue and cells can easily bounce back from the damage caused by alkylating agents, but the MIT team hypothesized that cells in inflamed tissue would show more damage from the chemicals, and their research supported their hypothesis. Tissues which were already dealing with inflammation and attempting to heal through

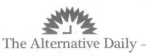

cell division showed much greater rates of mutation when exposed to the alkylating chemicals.

In a nutshell, this strongly suggests that individuals with inflammatory conditions are more susceptible to damage caused by carcinogens in the environment or food supply. This finding also extends to anyone with rapidly dividing cells, such as young children, developing embryos or those healing from injury or disease.

Similarly, irritating substances that originate inside the body, such as stomach acid and fecal bile acids, may lead to the development of cancer through an inflammatory mechanism. For example, chronic acid reflux exposes the tissue inside the esophagus to stomach acid, which causes inflammation. Over time, this can result in the same process of cell damage, mutation and cancer growth.

Other external substances can also cause a problem. Cigarette smoke, benzene, silica dust and asbestos are just a few examples of chemicals which can become lodged in tissues and cannot be cleared by the immune system. They can irritate the surrounding area, starting the familiar inflammatory cascade which can go wrong and veer down the cancerous route.

Finally, alcohol has been strongly implicated in causing inflammation in the liver, which can lead to tissue damage called liver cirrhosis, and ultimately hepatocarcinoma (liver cancer).

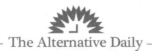

People with microbial conditions are more predisposed to cancer

Cancers can also be triggered by infectious agents. For example, the bacteria *Helicobacter pylori (H. pylori)* can double the risk for stomach cancer, and the same goes for hepatitis B or C viruses and liver cancer. A 2002 study published in the journal *Oncology* even goes so far as to say, "It seems that any parasitic infection that persists or recurs over many years can predispose to cancer. Thus, bacterial, viral, and parasitic infections can all lead to cancer if left unchecked." Therefore, it's not entirely surprising that some experts estimate that 15 percent of worldwide cancers may be due to microbial infections.

H. pylori is one of the more thoroughly studied microbial varieties. It has been observed that this infection causes inflammation of the mucosal tissues in the gut with an influx of immune cells such as lymphocytes, plasma cells, and neutrophils. Even despite the formidable attack put forth by the immune system, it's common for *H. pylori* infections to persist for decades, causing a twofold risk of developing stomach cancer, officially known as gastric adenocarcinoma.

Future research aims to determine whether treating the *H. pylori* infection with antibiotics succeeds in reducing the subsequent increased cancer risk. However, the risk of increasing susceptibility to further microbial infections by impairing the microbiome with antibiotics is an important consideration.

Parasitic and viral infections have also been strongly implicated in contributing to the development of various types of cancer. The following are a few examples:

- **Epstein-Barr virus:** Associated with B-cell non-Hodgkin's lymphoma.

- **Human immunodeficiency virus (HIV):** Predisposes the patient to non-Hodgkin's lymphoma, squamous cell carcinoma and Kaposi's sarcoma.

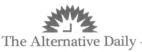

◆ **Schistosomiasis:** This parasitic infection linked to contaminated water supplies may lead to increased risk of bladder, liver, rectal and spleen cancers.

◆ **Liver flukes:** Parasites caught from eating raw fish can infect the bile duct and lead to a type of cancer called cholangiocarcinoma.

◆ **Human papillomavirus (HPV):** Associated with increased risk of cervical cancer, although this link requires further investigation.

At present, it is unclear whether viral infections contribute to the development of cancer by causing a chronic inflammatory environment in the infected area, by directly transforming the cells infected by the virus, or both. In any case, other studies support the hypothesis put forth by the MIT researchers mentioned earlier, where viruses induce tissue damage followed by a state of increased cell division and proliferation in an effort to make repairs, leaving these cells vulnerable to DNA damage and mutation.

Genetic factors at play

Although certain types of cancer can seem to run in families, only about five to ten percent of cancers result directly from gene defects or mutations being passed down the generations. However, since so many other factors can contribute to the

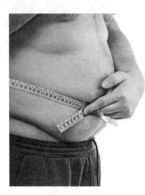

development of cancer, it stands to reason that family members may end up with similar illnesses. This could be through direct influencers such as asbestos in the family home causing lung inflammation, or an intestinal parasite that is passed around the family.

Common lifestyle factors can also contribute to the tendency to develop certain types of cancer. For example, family members may share a tendency toward colitis because of a

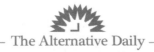

The Alternative Daily

common poor diet, may all have a similar excessive drinking habit, or perhaps tend to stress too much over the little things and develop inflammation as a result.

In this way, we can see that even though cancer itself may not be passed down, a family may share genetic tendencies in the way they react to inflammatory conditions. Researchers working with animal models, such as different species of mice, have found that certain strains exhibit much higher tendencies to develop tumors after exposure to inflammatory conditions and carcinogens.

Specific strains have been observed reacting to particular inflammatory chemicals by developing tumors, while other strains remained consistently resistant to cancer. This could explain why some people end up with cancer and others do not, even when they are exposed to similar adverse conditions such as smoking or chemical exposure.

Other risk factors for cancer

Besides inflammatory diseases, chemical exposure and genetics, there are a number of other factors which could play into a person's risk for developing cancer.

Age is one factor. Although this is absolutely not a certainty, there is a greater chance of older people being diagnosed, simply because many cancers can take decades to develop. This is tied to the likelihood of chronic inflammatory conditions and generally reduced immune function which go along with advancing age. However, some cancers form very quickly, so cancer can be found in people of any age.

Obesity contributes to the risk of cancer, and can also be considered an inflammatory pathway. People who are extremely overweight tend to carry systemic inflammation and extra fat around their organs. They also generally have dysfunctional hormonal and metabolic systems. All of this can add up to impaired immunity and cell function, potentially leading to cancer.

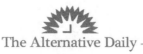

Sun exposure is another factor which can cause inflammation and gene mutation, which may result in skin cancer.

Even though these risk factors aren't directly considered inflammatory, it's clear to see that inflammation is the mechanism by which they become cancer risk factors.

Finally, the use of certain drugs and medical treatments can increase cancer risk. Some examples include oral contraceptives, menopause-related hormone replacement therapies, diethylstilbestrol (DES), Tamoxifen (a breast cancer drug), testosterone and other male hormones, radiation therapy and certain chemotherapy drugs (the alkylating agents referred to earlier). Some cancer drugs can actually contribute to the risk of a patient developing additional cancers in future years.

Issues with cancer drugs

With all of these risk factors for cancer, nearly all of us carry at least one. It's no surprise then that many people in First World countries will have some type of cancer in their lifetime. All of these cancer cases need treatment, and there are many drugs available. But do they really work, and are they worth the physical, mental and financial price?

Unfortunately, the "pill for an ill" mindset still prevails with many people today, and adopting a healthy preventative lifestyle is considered difficult, inconvenient and expensive. What many people don't know is that cancer treatments come with many risks, side effects and costs of their own.

To start with, many of the body's soft tissues, including the mouth and digestive tract, are made up of mucosal cells which are more sensitive to chemotherapy and radiation therapy. This means that a variety of problems can arise with these treatments, including mouth sores, ulcers, herpes infection and thrush or candida yeast overgrowth.

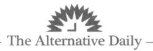

Keep in mind that, as we have been discussing, inflammation and infections in these tissues can play a role in contributing to cancer in the first place.

Similarly, within the digestive tract, diarrhea, constipation, nausea and vomiting are common side effects of chemotherapy. Patients being prepared for chemo treatment are usually given antinausea drugs in advance, but these can have side effects of their own, including lockjaw, confusion, headache, constipation and insomnia. Any number of drugs may be given to treat diarrhea and constipation, including narcotic analgesics (which require additional bowel therapy afterward to reinstate normal bowel functioning), morphine or oxycodone. These are all heavy drugs which exhibit a toxifying effect on the body, and especially the liver.

Besides drug side effects, cancer treatments can have devastating effects on other bodily tissues. This is because most of the treatments available today do not target cancer cells specifically, and run the risk of damaging other rapidly dividing cells as well. These include bone marrow cells, which are responsible for the production of red and white blood

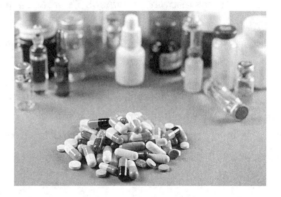

cells and platelets. A deficiency in these types of cells can cause bone pain, abnormal bleeding and increased vulnerability to infections. Additional treatments and even blood transfusions may be required in order to bring levels back to normal. It's easy to imagine that the impaired circulatory and immune function incited by these treatments could lead to a downward spiral toward other illnesses or cancers.

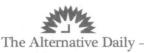

Other collateral damage of cancer treatments can include bladder or urinary toxicity, cardiac (heart) toxicity, hypersensitivity, allergic reactions, a number of different skin reactions, premature menopause, low sperm count and infertility. Many people who have undergone chemotherapy also report that they experience lethargy, fatigue, forgetfulness and impaired cognitive ability for months or even years following treatment.

A recent study published in the journal *Brain, Behavior and Immunity* pointed out that chemotherapy leaves an epigenetic imprint in the DNA of the white blood cells of breast cancer patients. Epigenetic settings act as switches which tell genes to turn on or off—in this study, the imprint left by chemotherapy ignited an inflammatory response for up to six months following treatment. The result is manifested similarly to the inflammatory reaction we get to a flu, with body aches, fatigue and lethargy. According to the study, these inflammatory epigenetic effects are experienced by up to 30 percent of breast cancer survivors.

The authors remained unsure whether the change to the epigenetic status of the white blood cells was altered directly by chemotherapy treatment, or whether this was a result of an inflammatory response to tissue injury caused by chemotherapy. In any case, it's clear that the cancer treatment ignites an inflammatory cascade similar to that which can trigger cancer in the first place.

Clearly, there are many concerns tied to the use of cancer drugs and treatments, not to mention the high financial costs, which can be anywhere from 9,000 to 46,000 dollars per course of chemotherapy in the US, depending on the type of cancer. Drugs are also extremely pricey: of the 12 drugs approved by the FDA for cancer conditions in 2012, 11 were priced above 100,000 dollars for a year of treatment. One drug approved for metastatic melanoma, which only improves patient survival times by a maximum of 3.7 months, costs 120,000 dollars for just four doses. Additional drugs used for the

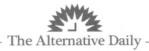

treatment of side effects can cost 35 dollars per one milligram tablet, or 300 dollars for a single injection.

Regardless of whether an individual can afford these considerable expenses, the cost to society should also be taken into account. For example, the WHO predicts that developing nations will struggle to provide the resources necessary to manage cancer in coming years. Also, insurance premiums will have to be increased in order to cover the unpredictable and wide-ranging costs. Many drugs are used for "off-label" indications. This means a drug is prescribed for an unapproved indication—one that is not included in its FDA-approved packaging label. While not illegal, off-label use often occurs with negligible supporting clinical data. Therefore, the cost to society could be carried needlessly for uses that were not prescribed and may not be effective.

Luckily, affordable holistic prevention and treatment options are available, and are being backed by increasing amounts of research.

Prevention is key: What you can do now to reduce your risk

Interestingly, the 2014 WHO World Cancer Report suggested that about half of all cancers were preventable through lifestyle factors such as smoking, alcohol consumption, diet and exercise, improved screening programs and vaccinations. This reinforces the fact that taking steps to prevent cancer by adopting a healthy lifestyle is crucially important.

Lung cancer remains the most commonly diagnosed type, at 1.8 million cases per year, or 13 percent of total diagnoses. Experts say that 80 to 90 percent of these cases could be prevented simply by quitting smoking.

Bevin Engelward, a professor of biological engineering at MIT, believes toxins (such as certain foods and chemicals) can lead to DNA damage and should be avoided. He says that recent research confirms there are also other preventative strategies which can be undertaken to slow or halt the progression of cancer. One example is avoiding exposure to environmental factors, which can be problematic.

On the flip side of that coin, we find a long list of holistic preventive practices which can undo damage and prevent further inflammatory episodes.

The following are some practical steps that you can integrate into your daily life, one by one, on your own. If you are experiencing symptoms of moderate to severe inflammation, or can't shake off a chronic condition, seeking the assistance of a holistic-minded health-care professional that you trust is advised.

Reduce chemical exposure

As we have mentioned, many types of cancer are associated with developed, industrialized nations and the chemical exposure that comes along with this type of society. Many people are exposed to hazardous chemicals in the workplace or via the daily use of consumer products that damage the body's innate balance and cause inflammation.

Heavy metals top the list of things to avoid. Some of the most common offenders are lead piping, mercury dental fillings and the consumption of certain fish. Ensure that you are not consuming water that has been piped through lead and have mercury fillings removed and replaced with safe ones by a holistic dentist. Choose only safe species of fish, such as wild-caught Pacific and Alaskan salmon, or small types such as sardines and herring, which are less likely to accumulate mercury.

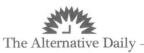

Some sources of groundwater can also contain trace amounts of heavy metals, which accumulate over time, so it may be helpful to have your home's water system tested. Heavy metal contamination is a significant source of inflammation. It is therefore worth the effort to investigate and avoid exposure.

Plastics also cause issues in the body. Their molecular structure can be similar to human hormones, which act as vital signalers in all systems throughout the body. It's easy to imagine how interfering with these systems would result in widespread toxicity and inflammation. Breaking up with plastic will be one of the best things you can do for yourself and your family. Use glass and stainless steel food containers whenever possible. Silicone is considered safe for items that do not come into direct contact with food, but do not use it for extreme temperature applications such as freezing or baking.

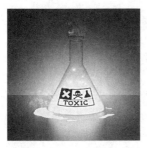

Following in the line of avoiding chemical exposure, have you considered the toxic load of your household cleaning and personal toiletry products? While we purchase these things without a second thought and use them in our immediate environment and on our bodies daily, they actually contain a frightening amount of chemicals, which have far-reaching effects on bodily systems.

Never fear: it's easy to replace these items with nontoxic alternatives, which are often more affordable, as well. Coconut oil, baking soda and vinegar will perform the vast majority of tasks you've ever done around the home! And if you want a nice scent, feel free to use a few drops of lemon essential oil in your cleaning products.

Consume less alcohol and tobacco

This one is a bit of a no-brainer. While complete abstinence is not mandatory in the case of alcohol, using these toxic and inflammatory substances should be kept to a

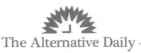

minimum. The connections to lung and liver cancer are extremely well established in relation to heavy smoking or drinking, so while it may be difficult to give up these habits, the payoff in terms of cancer prevention is a considerable one!

Address chronic inflammatory conditions

As we've discussed, chronic inflammatory conditions are major contributors to the development of cancer. Many people are unable or unwilling to expend the effort to resolve these conditions, which can stick around for decades.

Speak with a holistic health or functional medicine practitioner to learn the best way to resolve your particular condition. Using pharmaceuticals (such as antibiotics to resolve an *H. pylori* infection, or special mouthwash for gum disease) usually only addresses the symptoms and does not fix the root cause.

Avoid parasites and mold

Fungal and parasitic organisms, like bacteria and viruses, can wreak havoc in the human body. Parasites are more common than we think—some estimates indicate that one in three Americans is living with a parasite.

Taking precautions when you travel to foreign countries and getting the family pets checked often are good strategies for avoiding infection by a parasite.

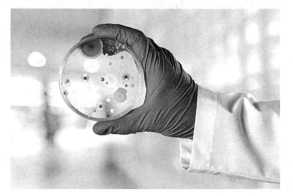

Mold can similarly cause damage and inflammation, even in the brain! Ensuring that your home is mold-free is very important for the health

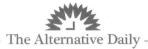

of your family. Basements, attics and cottages can be hotbeds for mold. Regular maintenance and waterproofing can help reduce moisture. If there is an existing problem, professional mold removal is prudent.

Anti-inflammatory foods

An increasing body of research supports the role of a healthy, whole-foods diet in the fight against cancer. We know that eating the right foods can put out inflammatory fires and encourage proper cell function, while other foods can do the exact opposite. You'll find more in-depth information about "good and bad foods" in Chapter 12 of this book.

First, the ones to avoid. In general, this group includes white and brown foods. The forbidden white foods are sugar, flour (bread, pasta, etc.) and trans fats such as shortening or hydrogenated oils. In the brown group, we have deep-fried junk, soda, too much caffeine and lifeless fast food. Also, drop any foods that may cause an allergic or inflammatory response for you, personally. Gluten, commercial dairy products, corn, soy and some nuts are common culprits. These items make you fat, sick, tired and inflamed. Just say "no, thank you!"

Instead, we want to stick with lots of foods from the following healthy groups:

Colorful fruits and vegetables

Have you heard the phrase "eat the rainbow?" We're not talking about colorful candy, but rather the bountiful fresh foods that nature provides. Think red strawberries, watermelon and currants, orange peppers, carrots and squash, yellow lemons, zucchini and apples, 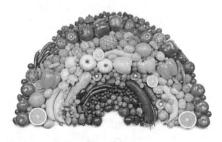 green spinach, cucumber and fennel, and blue eggplant, currants and blueberries.

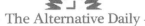

All of these vibrant foods are packed with phytochemicals (plant nutrients) and antioxidants which help maintain healthy cell function and clean up free radical damage. This is what prevents cells from malfunctioning, mutating and potentially becoming cancerous.

One serving of fruit and vegetables is just half a cup, which is no more than a small handful, so it's easy to pack in many servings each day. Try to incorporate at least 20 to 30 different vegetables into your diet over the span of a week.

A quick note of caution: there is a group of vegetables called nightshades which may cause an inflammatory and autoimmune response in some people. These include tomatoes, peppers and eggplant, amongst others. Nightshades are a common contributor to autoimmune conditions such as arthritis and multiple sclerosis. If this is an issue for you, there are many, many other wonderful fresh fruits and vegetables to eat instead. If you are unsure whether nightshades affect you, talk to a health professional you trust.

Healthy fats

Contrary to the waning "fat-free craze," fats are one of the most important anti-inflammatory foods you can eat! Fats allow for healthy brain function and cell repair, as well as the absorption of many vitamins which are only soluble in fat. They also provide the raw materials for hormones (the body's signalers and messengers). They are a great source of fuel and long-lasting energy, and do not usually get stored as body fat (which is counter-intuitive, but true).

Which fats are best to eat? Good plant sources include nuts and seeds, and cold-pressed minimally-processed nut and seed oils. Go for avocados and avocado oil, coconut and coconut oil, walnuts and walnut oil, ground flaxseed, pumpkin seeds and sesame seeds.

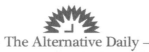

Animal-based healthy fats must come from wild and pastured sources. Butter and other full-fat dairy products from pastured cows are packed with nutrients, as are eggs, lard and tallow from naturally-raised animals. Wild-caught cold-water fish contain the much sought-after omega-3 fatty acids, which are notoriously lacking in our modern diets. Choose species such as wild salmon, mackerel, sardines and herring.

Some fats should definitely be avoided. These are generally the man-made and industrially processed ones. Avoid anything hydrogenated, as well as vegetable oils made with high heat, pressure and solvents, such as corn, soybean, cottonseed and sunflower oils. Fats from factory-farmed animals may also be toxic.

Clean protein

Along the lines of the above section on fats, animal protein should also be obtained from wild or pastured, organic, naturally-cultivated sources. The nutrient and chemical makeup of healthy animals is entirely different, and far better for us, than those raised in confinement with drugs, engineered feed and growth

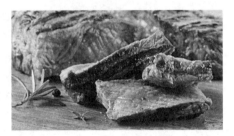

agents. Spending a little bit of extra effort and resources on seeking out quality meat, eggs and fish will pay off in the anti-inflammatory nourishment your body receives.

Fermented and cultured foods

Have you heard of kombucha, kefir or sauerkraut? These foods are some of the oldest in the world, yet some of the newest on the modern health scene. As we discussed earlier in this book, scientists, and the general public, are realizing that bacteria are a major contributor to human health, and consuming beneficial probiotics is an important part of an anti-cancer / anti-inflammatory diet. Making your own fermented and cultured

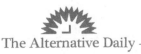

foods is easy and rewarding, but if you're buying commercially produced ones, ensure that they are unpasteurized and contain minimal ingredients. Try to consume at least two to three tablespoons of probiotic foods each day!

Natural remedies that calm inflammation

As Hippocrates said long ago, "Let food be thy medicine." This wisdom stands true today, where most of nature's anti-inflammatory remedies are those we put on our plate. However, there are some other valuable healing substances that we can use as natural medicines or supplements, as well. These whole, unprocessed remedies can often be more effective than man-made pharmaceuticals, because they interact with the body in an intelligent fashion.

According to a professor of medicine and neurology from the University of California, Los Angeles, "While anti-inflammatory drugs usually block a single target molecule and reduce its activity dramatically, natural anti-inflammatories gently tweak a broader range of inflammatory compounds. You'll get greater safety and efficacy reducing five inflammatory mediators by 30 percent than by reducing one by 100 percent."

The following are a few natural remedies to consider incorporating into your preventative regime. To be safe, consult a health professional you trust before beginning a regimen with any of these remedies.

Herbs and spices

It's time to stock up your pantry with anti-inflammatory herbs and spices! Whether you add them to recipes, mix them into DIY toiletry products or consume them as supplements, these potent natural remedies have a lot to offer.

Rosemary, with its active ingredient rosmarinic acid, is one of the best cancer-fighting herbs out there, with studies showing it can kill up to 93 percent of cervical cancer cells.

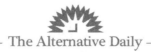

Garlic is also a perennial immune-booster, and may be highly effective for many chronic or acute conditions. Let freshly chopped garlic sit for 10 minutes before adding it to recipes to allow the active ingredient, allicin, to multiply several times over.

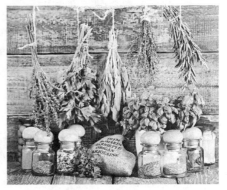

Others to add to your regimen include spices such as turmeric, chilli pepper, ginger, cumin and black pepper.

Herbs are also a goldmine of antioxidants, nutrients and blood-cleansing compounds. Try basil, coriander, dill, fennel, oregano and sage. If you can grow or buy fresh herbs, try storing them in the freezer in the form of ice cubes, which can be easily added to any smoothie, soup or stir-fry.

Essential oils

Did you know that essential oils are the original medicine? When you walk through a pine forest or peel an orange, you are smelling the volatile oils emitted by those plants. Essential oils are simply potent extracts made by the gentle pressing or distillation of medicinal plants. This is a great way to harness the amazing remedies hidden within nature's bounty. This simple form of medicine has been used for millennia, and is also available today. When shopping for essential oils, be sure to seek out good-quality therapeutic-grade products.

A number of essential oils have been studied for their cancer-fighting and anti-inflammatory power. Frankincense essential oil, distilled from the resin of the boswellia tree, is one of the best overall inflammation fighters, helping to shut down cell abnormalities and soothe tissues. Lavender essential oil is excellent for healing

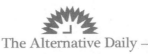

both the body and a stressed or anxious mind. Cinnamon, oregano and clove oils are some of the best choices for fighting chronic fungal or bacterial infections, which would otherwise keep that dangerous inflammatory fire burning.

Herbal teas

While essential oils are highly potent extracts, teas are a gentler form of plant medicine, and a safe and effective way to consume beneficial anti-inflammatory and immune-supportive compounds. Green tea in particular has received much praise for its ability to protect cells from free radical damage, one of the first factors that can lead to cancer.

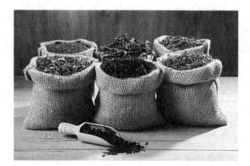

Other types of tea can contribute to the prevention of cancer indirectly, by providing support to body systems and relieving stress. For example, chamomile tea is excellent for calming the stress response (which we know is a problematic source of inflammation), and peppermint tea can improve digestion (allowing for the absorption of valuable anticancer nutrients from your food).

Medicinal teas made from mushrooms such as chaga and reishi can also help the body adapt to stress and fend off free radical damage and inflammation.

Lifestyle practices to fight inflammation

Your mental state and everyday habits have a significant impact on the inflammatory load your body carries. Let's take a look at a few of these.

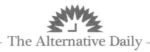

Stress relief

It is estimated that 95 percent of doctor visits today are related to chronic stress, so this is clearly a force to be reckoned with. It's important to recognize that stress is not an absolute—it's largely about the way you choose to react to challenges in your life. For example, a snow storm may bring misery and inconvenience to some, while others choose to see it as an opportunity for enjoyable hibernation and recreation!

The idea that emotion and state of mind can be manifested as disease may seem too "out there" for many. However, it is certainly worth consideration. In a nutshell, a chronic sense of stress engages the body's sympathetic nervous system, which fires up stress-related hormones like cortisol and adrenaline, and shuts down "non-essential" processes like digestion, cellular maintenance, immunity and fertility. The stress response is by and large an inflammatory mechanism, whereby the body and mind are on high alert and little (if any) healing is achieved. With many of us living in a constant state of fight-or-flight, it's no surprise that cancer grows.

Therefore, it is vital to engage in self-care practices to lower the stress that arises in modern life. Time spent in nature, yoga, meditation, playing games with family and friends, making music or art and breathing exercises are excellent ways to quiet the stress response and encourage the body's natural healing processes. For more information about stress and inflammation, see Chapter 13 of this book.

Adequate rest

Sleep is also a vital part of avoiding inflammation and cancer. During good quality sleep, various anabolic processes are carried out, whereby the body builds and repairs tissues and disposes of damaged cells and waste materials.

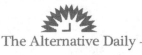

For this restful, healing sleep to occur, melatonin production must be encouraged. Unfortunately, using electronic devices and living in artificial light in the evenings shuts down the production of this vital sleep-promoting and cancer-fighting substance.

You can encourage melatonin production in preparation for sleep by using low-blue lights or candles in your home after dark, and wearing yellow or orange glasses, particularly when using electronic devices or watching TV. Shutting off all electronics an hour before bed is also a smart idea.

Exercise

Moving your body is important for so many reasons, particularly to fight inflammation, degeneration and cancer. At its most basic, exercise promotes blood and lymph fluid circulation, which help to move oxygen and nutrients around the body and discard damaged cells and waste products.

Physical activity also reduces stress and improves sleep. Human growth hormone is produced when you exercise, which facilitates growth and repair of healthy tissue.

Many recent studies support the premise that moderate, regular exercise is an effective tool against inflammation, and ultimately, cancer. Beneficial side effects include flexibility, youthfulness and a fit figure!

You don't need an expensive gym membership or a special outfit—just move! There are many bodyweight routines you can do on the rug in the living room in your pajamas, so there really is no excuse. You can start a regular exercise routine, or you can just incorporate enjoyable play and movement into your leisure time or

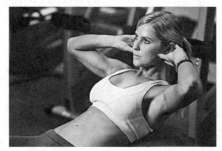

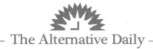

The Alternative Daily

errands. Go for a walk after dinner, throw a Frisbee in the park, or ride a bike to the supermarket.

For more in-depth information about exercise and inflammation, see Chapter 14.

Sunlight

You are probably familiar with the concept of sunlight facilitating vitamin D production. Vitamin D plays an important role in supporting the immune system to fight inflammation and potential cancerous cells. Ensure that you get at least 30 minutes of sun exposure on your face and arms, whenever the season allows! When it's not possible 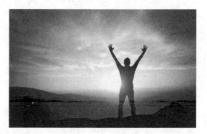 to get natural vitamin D, using a vitamin D3 supplement (at least 1,000 IU per day with research showing little to no downsides of taking 4,000 IUs per day) is helpful and safe for most people. Getting vitamin D from a high quality cod liver oil is also an excellent option.

Avoid the use of pharmaceuticals whenever possible

With all of the holistic health practices described above, the use of pharmaceutical drugs should be eliminated whenever possible. Many pharmaceutical drugs may quell symptoms, but cause a considerable amount of collateral damage in the process. As the old saying goes, "an ounce of prevention is worth a pound of cure." Using holistic health practices to keep your body healthy is well worth the effort to avoid the toxicity and even residual inflammation caused by medications. Of course, in the case of an emergency, or a serious health issue, medication may become necessary. However, it's best not to turn to pharmaceutical options unless you really have to.

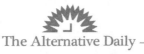

Unfortunately, even with our best prevention efforts, cancer may still strike. If you or someone you know does happen to be diagnosed, make sure to explore all of your treatment options thoroughly, keeping in mind that what's right for one person may not be right for another. Along with your doctor, it may be helpful to seek the advice of a reputable holistic health professional, as well, so that you have all the information at your disposal to make the treatment choice that's right for you.

Chapter Eleven
Arthritis: Red, Hot and Swollen

*D*id you know there is more than one type of arthritis? In addition to arthritis that attacks bones, there is also arthritis that attacks joints, arthritis that attacks the entire nervous system and even local types of arthritis such as carpal tunnel syndrome. All in all, there are over 20 types of arthritis.

In general, arthritis is divided into two main categories: arthritis of the tissues surrounding the joint (typically known as rheumatoid arthritis, or RA), and arthritis of the bones themselves (typically known as osteoarthritis, or OA). Many adults suffer from both RA and OA as they age. In addition to these two main categories, there are also numerous specific types of arthritis. The most common types are listed below:

Adult-onset Still's disease (AOSD): Adult-onset Still's disease is a form of arthritis that has many symptoms similar to rheumatoid arthritis, but it is a rarer form of the disease. Still's disease typically sets in during the adult years and affects just a few joints at first, but can spread throughout the entire body. In some cases, Still's disease lasts only a short time, but in other cases, it can trigger chronic arthritis symptoms.

Ankylosing spondylitis (AS): AS is a type of arthritis that is commonly felt in the back, buttocks, hips and lower spine. This is a common form of arthritis that typically starts

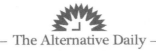

with small symptoms that gradually worsen over time. In many cases, people with AS are never officially diagnosed, as they just feel the pain is a symptom of aging that will never get better.

Bursitis: Bursitis is a type of temporary arthritis that affects the bursa sac that acts as a cushion between bones and muscles. If the bursa sac is damaged from overuse, the area will become inflamed and sore. Treatment is typically to avoid using the joint as much as possible until the sac has time to heal. "Tennis elbow" is a common form of bursitis arthritis.

Calcium pyrophosphate dihydrate crystal deposition disease (CPPD): CPPD is a condition where crystal deposits form on the joints. The crystal deposits irritate the joint, which causes inflammation and joint pain typical of arthritis. CPPD is similar to gout, rheumatoid arthritis and osteoarthritis.

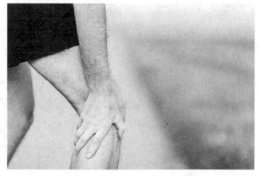

Chondromalacia patella (CP): CP is a type of knee-specific arthritis that occurs from overuse of the joint. This condition causes general pain and stiffness combined with a "grinding" feeling in the knees. CP is commonly seen in athletes, manual laborers and other individuals who are highly active. When the joint is rested, the pain goes away.

Degenerative disc disease (DDD): DDD is a back-specific form of osteoarthritis that is caused by the vertebrae in the back degenerating. Over time, everyone's vertebrae deteriorate, but in some people, the bones break down faster and cause more pain. When the pain is unrelated to other issues, it is typically diagnosed as DDD.

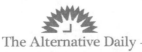

Gout: Gout is a form of arthritis that affects the joints, and is caused by elevated levels of uric acid in the body. Obesity, excessive alcohol use and an underactive thyroid can all cause uric acid levels to rise. Gout typically affects men more than women, and is usually identified by intense pain and swelling in one of the big toes, which spreads to other locations.

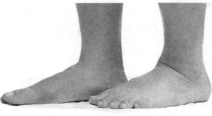

Infectious arthritis: Infectious arthritis is a type of arthritis brought on by an infection. It is usually temporary, and symptoms fade when the original infection heals. Common infections that trigger infectious arthritis include Lyme disease, measles, mumps, fifth disease and rheumatic fever. Infectious arthritis is typically caused by bacterial infections.

Inflammatory arthritis: Inflammatory arthritis is a type of arthritis directly caused by excessive levels of inflammation in the joints. Inflammatory arthritis is the larger grouping for specific inflammatory forms of arthritis such as rheumatoid arthritis and ankylosing spondylitis.

Juvenile idiopathic arthritis (JIA): JIA is a form of autoimmune arthritis where the immune system attacks the tissues surrounding the joints. This causes pain in children and is difficult to treat. The precise cause of JIA is unknown, and it is estimated to affect about 300,000 children in the United States.

Mixed connective tissue disease (MCTD): MCTD is a type of joint-related inflammation that mimics symptoms of several arthritis-related conditions. MCTD is an autoimmune disorder where the body attacks connective tissues in the joints.

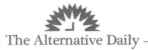

Osteoarthritis (OA): OA is the most common form of arthritis today and is known as the "wear and tear" form of arthritis. OA pain occurs from the tissues and bones breaking down due to aging. Obesity is one significant risk factor for developing OA.

Palindromic rheumatism (PR): PR is a form of inflammatory arthritis that comes and goes. Symptoms will appear for several days in a row, then the patient will feel fine for several additional days or weeks. In about 50 percent of cases, PR develops into full-blown rheumatoid arthritis as a person ages.

Reactive arthritis: Reactive arthritis is a form of the disease that attacks the joints during a period of infection. It only occurs when a bacterial infection enters the bloodstream.

Rheumatoid arthritis (RA): RA is the second most-common form of arthritis. RA occurs when the immune system attacks healthy cells and tissues surrounding the joints, causing swelling and pain. This can result in stiffness, which can make it difficult to function normally. Some health experts believe RA is preventable and reversible, while others do not.

Spinal stenosis: Spinal stenosis is a form of osteoarthritis where the spine narrows in specific areas of the back. When this occurs, it places additional pressure on the spine, causing pain and inflammation. In severe cases, spinal stenosis can cause severe nerve pain and damage if the spine presses against a nerve in the back.

What causes arthritis?

The medical industry does not yet have a clear explanation for what causes the different forms of arthritis to appear. However, there are a few theories on what may trigger or cause arthritis:

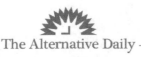

Inflammation: Many forms of arthritis are triggered or worsened by excessive inflammation in the body. Chronic inflammation may trigger some forms of arthritis, and could even be behind some of the autoimmune forms of arthritis.

Overuse: Many of the bone-related arthritis types are caused by overuse. Both overuse in short bursts and overuse over time will increase the risk of developing arthritis.

Trauma: A broken bone or even a bad sprain may lead to the development of arthritis in the years following the injury. Injuries are also more likely to lead to the faster breakdown of the joints, which can lead to osteoarthritis.

Infections: Several types of arthritis are tied to bacterial infections. Bacterial infections trigger whole-body joint pain and immune responses, which typically fade when the infection disappears, but not all the time.

Autoimmune imbalances: Scientists and health experts are not entirely certain what causes autoimmune diseases to pop up, but if your body has an autoimmune problem, you are more likely to have autoimmune-related arthritis symptoms. A body of research suggests that autoimmune problems may be affected by diet and chronic inflammation.

The role of inflammation

Inflammation and arthritis appear to have significant links, although scientists are just starting to figure out the connection. Some researchers theorize that elevated levels of inflammation can trigger an overactive immune response in the body, which could trigger arthritis symptoms.

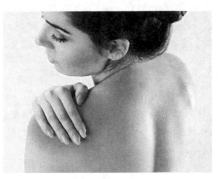

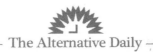

The Alternative Daily

Several forms of arthritis, including the common RA, are considered autoimmune diseases. Inflammation is often one of the first signs of an autoimmune disorder. If inflammation and arthritis are linked, then it follows that by reducing inflammation, you may be able to reduce your arthritis symptoms.

The bacteria connection

New research suggests that an intestinal bacterial imbalance may cause some cases of autoimmune disease, such as arthritis. A 2013 study published in *eLife* found that most study participants with RA had an increase in a type of bacteria known as *Prevotella copri*. Additionally, the same study participants had lower levels of bacteria commonly associated with a stronger immune system.

Researchers theorize that some of the autoimmune diseases we see today, such as RA, may be caused by an imbalance of the right bacteria in the intestines. Bacteria levels and the immune system can be adjusted by making different, and smarter, lifestyle choices, such as adopting a whole, nutritious diet.

Joint pain triggers

According to research, joint pain can be controlled through a series of lifestyle changes. The following is a list of common triggers for joint pain. By eliminating these triggers, it is possible to reduce or even eliminate many symptoms of rheumatoid arthritis, and even some symptoms of osteoarthritis.

Uric acid

An excess of uric acid in the body leads to a form of arthritis known as gout. Gout used to be an extremely common form of arthritis, but today, it is not as common as osteoarthritis and rheumatoid arthritis. Gout normally starts as extreme joint pain,

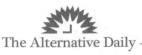

swelling, and sensitivity in one of the big toes, but over time, it spreads to the rest of the joints in the body.

The following is a list of factors that may raise uric acid levels in the body:

Excess weight: If you are overweight, you are more likely to have high uric acid levels. Uric acid is produced during the breakdown and turnover of cells, and when you are overweight, there are simply more cells to turn over. This increases your uric acid concentrations significantly, and the more you weigh, the higher your uric acid levels are.

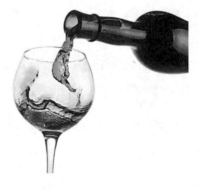

Alcohol abuse: Alcohol interferes with the body's ability to remove uric acid from the body. If you drink in moderation this is not a problem, because when you stop drinking the body can take care of excessive levels of uric acid. However, when you constantly drink or binge drink on a regular basis, your body cannot eliminate uric acid, which can cause problems and elevated levels of uric acid.

A diet rich in purines: A purine is a type of chemical, found in certain foods, which converts to uric acid in the body. This makes the consumption of purines undesirable for individuals with gout and other forms of arthritis. High levels of purines are found in the following foods:

- Dried legumes
- Anchovies
- Kidneys
- Game meat

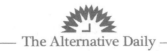

- Asparagus
- Sardines
- Herring
- Liver
- Mackerel
- Scallops

Medical issues: A few medical conditions can contribute to high levels of uric acid, including high blood pressure, an underactive thyroid, kidney problems, cancer, psoriasis and hemolytic anemia.

Trigger foods

Research suggests that certain foods can play a role in joint pain. According to the Arthritis Foundation, the following are a few of the foods that may lead to inflammation in the body and potentially trigger RA symptoms:

Sugar: According to the *American Journal of Clinical Nutrition,* sugar raises cytokine levels in the body, which triggers inflammation. As we discussed previously, all forms of sugar can trigger inflammation, regardless of the source or the name of the sugar.

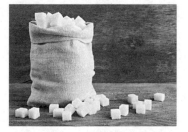

Trans fats: Trans fats are in nearly all forms of processed foods. Any food with the label of partially hydrogenated oil contains harmful trans fats. Trans fats are unusable by the body, but the body often confuses them for usable fats. When the body tries to

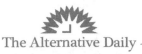

use this type of fat, it triggers an inflammatory response as it works harder to eliminate the dangerous fat. Trans fats are one of the most inflammatory foods we eat today.

Omega-6 fats: Omega-6 fats are healthy when eaten in small amounts, but when you consume too many, the fats are detrimental to your body and encourage excessive inflammation. Omega-6 fats are found in corn oil, sunflower oil, safflower oil, canola oil, peanut oil, grape seed oil and almost any form of vegetable oil. In general, your ratio of omega-6s to omega-3s should be about 3 to 1. However, many Americans diet is in a ratio of 25 to 1, which has a significant inflammatory effect on the body.

Casein and gluten: Casein is a protein found in dairy products that is difficult for some people to break down. Gluten is another protein that is difficult for the body to process. If you are sensitive to dairy and/or gluten, you may be worsening your inflammation by continuing to eat these substances on a regular basis.

Smoking

Smoking is extremely bad for the body. It damages cells in the lungs and throughout the body, increasing the risk of a whole host of other problems. One of the side effects of chronic smoking is constant inflammation, which can trigger joint pain.

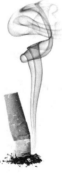

High-impact exercise

Some forms of exercise are hard on the joints, which can lead to the development of arthritis. Usually the effects are temporary and disappear when the activity stops. However, if you have OA or RA, high-impact exercise could make symptoms worse.

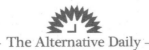

Inactive lifestyle

On the other hand, if you are too sedentary you will also have a higher chance of joint pain symptoms. A study of over 5,000 elderly patients with arthritis, conducted by the Feinberg School of Medicine, found that individuals who did not exercise on a regular basis increased their risk of worsening arthritis by 200 percent. Over two years, individuals who did not exercise saw their arthritis symptoms worsen by 14 percent.

Stress

A 2009 study conducted by the CDC found that individuals who had higher levels of daily stress were more likely to have raised levels of inflammation, and consequently, arthritis symptoms.

Obesity

The link between obesity and arthritis is clear. Not only does obesity raise uric acid levels in the blood, but it also increases generalized inflammation, potentially leading to an increase in arthritis symptoms.

Reduce your arthritis pain today

You don't have to live with arthritis pain forever. Although in some cases arthritis pain will always be present to some extent, you can greatly reduce your pain levels by reducing your total inflammation.

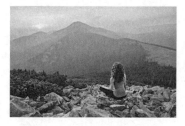

These simple lifestyle changes can make a big impact on your overall health and the severity of your arthritis symptoms. Implement these today and you'll likely start feeling better before you know it.

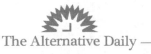

Exercise

Exercise helps ease pain in the joints, improves mobility, fights inflammation and reduces stress all at the same time. Low-impact exercise is ideal for individuals with arthritis, as high-impact exercise can make symptoms worse. Aim to exercise for about 30 minutes three to four times a week, and build up from there. You can start with something simple like walking or swimming and add in more difficult exercises as your health improves. The most important thing is to move regularly.

Stop smoking and drinking

Smoking and drinking both promote joint pain. If you suffer from arthritis, you can benefit your joint health by significantly reducing or completely eliminating smoking and drinking from your life. Limit alcohol consumption to no more than two drinks per week, and ditch the cigarettes—they aren't doing your body any favors.

Lose that weight

As we've discussed, obesity raises inflammation and arthritis pain levels. Do what you can to drop any excess weight that you may have, and your arthritis symptoms will likely start to lighten. The easiest and most effective way to lose weight is by implementing a healthy diet and exercising at least three to four times a week. Avoid fad diets, as this can lead to yo-yo weight gain, which is damaging to joints and your body's other systems.

Reduce stress

Stress is a huge factor in inflammation, as we'll discuss in further detail in Chapter 13. Stress can take over and cause a host of problems in the body, such as weight

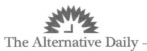

gain, insomnia, irritability, and a reduced immune system. Do your best to reduce your day-to-day stress levels to control some of the pain associated with arthritis. You can reduce stress in any of the following ways:

Create a relaxing nighttime routine: About an hour before bed, take time to relax. Try reading a book, taking a warm shower or bath, or drinking a cup of your favorite healthy beverage, such as chamomile tea. Try not to use electronics or phones during this time.

Meditate: Meditation can work wonders in relieving stress. If you are new to meditation, you may wish to attend a meditation session or browse the web for instructional videos. Alternatively, you can simply focus on guided imagery, or use this time to practice deep breathing exercises. Even just taking a few moments to breathe deeply can help reduce stress.

Sleep well: If you are not sleeping, then your body cannot effectively eliminate stress. The National Sleep Foundation recommends that adults get between seven and nine hours of quality sleep each night. If you create a nighttime routine as outlined above, you are setting the stage for healthy sleep habits that promote rest and relaxation. Ensuring you get adequate sleep will help fight inflammation.

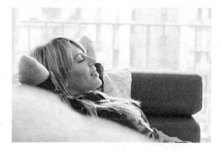

Eat your omega-3s

As mentioned, most Americans get far too little omega-3 fat in their diet. Omega-3s are found in foods such as fatty fish, flax seeds and chia seeds. The best way to adjust your balance of omega fats is to reduce consumption of omega-6 fats while increasing omega-3 fats.

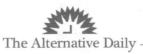

Balance your bacteria

The studies outlined in earlier sections suggest that bacteria can play a larger role in inflammation and arthritis than previously thought. Evidence suggests that the right balance of bacteria is extremely beneficial to overall health. If you suspect your bacteria levels may be out of balance, eat fermented foods several times a week in combination with a healthy diet, and add a high-quality probiotic supplement to your routine. Even if it doesn't help directly with pain, balanced bacteria levels will at the very least improve your digestion.

Treat pain with hot and cold therapy

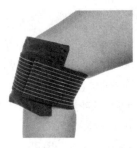

A combination of hot and cold therapy can help reduce the symptoms and flare-ups of arthritis. For joint pain, apply a cold pack to the sore joint for no more than 20 minutes at a time. To relieve stiffness, apply a hot pad for up to 20 minutes at a time. Use a heating pad at night to increase flexibility and reduce stiffness. Try a combination of hot and cold on particularly painful joints by applying a cold pack for five minutes and then switching to a hot pad for another five minutes. Repeat until pain and stiffness subsides.

Try alternative therapies

The Arthritis Foundation states that several alternative therapies for arthritis have been shown to have positive effects. Some of the most common alternative therapies are listed below:

Herbal supplements: A few herbs have been shown in scientific studies to have positive effects on inflammation. Turmeric is one excellent inflammation fighter, but

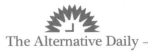

there are also other herbs that could be beneficial, including garlic, stinging nettle, boswellia, ginkgo biloba and devil's claw. Since herbs can be highly potent, it's a good idea to check with a health professional before beginning a regimen with them.

Acupuncture: According to the Arthritis Foundation, many patients with arthritis pain report relief after acupuncture sessions. Make sure your acupuncturist is qualified to work on joint pain before booking your appointment.

Physical therapy: Physical therapy works directly on your joints through massage and manipulation. In some cases, this can relieve some pain and stiffness associated with different forms of arthritis. Make sure your physical therapist is qualified to work with arthritis patients.

Chapter Twelve
Bad Food, Good Food

As we noted earlier, the rates of obesity and many chronic inflammatory illnesses are going up in the United States—in both adults and children. The funny thing is, we rarely look at our diets as the key to our health. Hippocrates said it best, "Let food be thy medicine and medicine be thy food."

Bad food

Even when we do assess the foods we eat— and most of us are at least somewhat aware of foods that are not good for us (that bag of cookies isn't winning any health prizes)—we often do not change our diets until disease is already upon us.

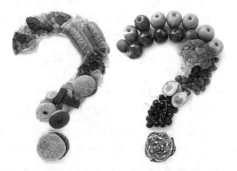

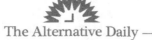

However we justify our food choices, the fact remains, the foods we put into our bodies each day have an enormous impact on our health. Think about it: the things you put into your mouth serve to fuel your body. It may sound incredibly simple, but it is an often-ignored notion.

It is because of the direct connection between the foods we eat and the state of our bodies that the Western diet is so dangerous. Laden with inflammation-causing foods, this diet, so prevalent in the U.S. and many other parts of the world, is destroying our bodies. As much as we'd like to point to other sources for the cause of our soaring chronic disease rates, we must first look at our diets in order to make a change for the better.

The following are the top foods that promote inflammation, muddle the body's immune system, and allow chronic illnesses to flourish. We've mentioned some of these before, but because they are so dangerous, they deserve a closer look.

Sugar

The head of Amsterdam's health service, Paul van der Velpen, recently wrote, "This may seem exaggerated and far-fetched, but sugar is the most dangerous drug of the times." Looking closely at how sugar works in the body, and its ill effects, this statement does not appear exaggerated at all.

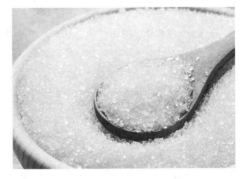

When we eat sugar, which is made up of glucose and fructose, the fructose that is not immediately used for energy is stored in the liver as fat. Not only can this promote weight gain and dangerous visceral fat, which coats vital organs, it may also lead to insulin resistance. The processing of fructose by the body also releases hydrogen peroxide within our cells, which can destroy them and contribute to accelerated aging.

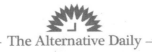

In 2011, a study published in the *American Journal of Clinical Nutrition* sought to determine the effects of sugar-sweetened beverages (abbreviated in the study as SSBs) on healthy young men. The factors tested were blood sugar, metabolism, cholesterol levels and signs of inflammation.

On their results, the study authors wrote:

"The present data show potentially harmful effects of low to moderate consumption of SSBs on markers of cardiovascular risk such as LDL particles, fasting glucose, and hs-CRP [C-reactive protein] within just 3 weeks in healthy young men, which is of particular significance for young consumers."

C-reactive protein is a known marker of inflammation, and research published in the *American Journal of Clinical Nutrition* has also found that processed sugars, such as those found in SSBs may contribute to the release of cytokines, messengers of inflammation.

What is especially frightening about the above-mentioned study is that low to moderate intake of sugary beverages had these effects—not just a high intake. Therefore, if we think that drinking soda and other sugary drinks in moderation is no big deal, it looks like we are just plain wrong.

Also, according to Dr. Nicholas Perricone, a dermatologist and nutritionist:

"Sugar suppresses the activity of our white blood cells, which makes us more susceptible to infectious disease (colds, the flu, and so forth) as well as cancer."

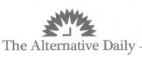

Wheat

It is well known that wheat—including whole wheat—can cause inflammation in individuals with celiac disease, which make up about one percent of the population. As we've discussed, in individuals with celiac disease, the body has an autoimmune reaction to gluten, a protein found in wheat, as well as in barley and rye.

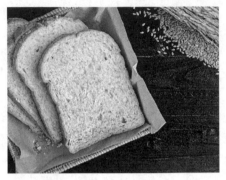

When a person with celiac disease consumes gluten, severe inflammation occurs, which can cause damage to the lining of the small intestine and a compromised ability to absorb nutrients. Although only one percent of the population is estimated to have full celiac disease, some health professionals hypothesize that potentially 30 to 40 percent of the global population may have some degree of gluten sensitivity, which is often overlooked.

However, what about those individuals who are not sensitive to gluten? The bad news is, wheat can cause inflammation in all of us, because it's not just the glutenous portion that is inflammatory. Wheat contains a complex carbohydrate called amylopectin A, which is easily digested by the body, and can cause blood sugar to rapidly spike.

This quick spike in blood sugar gives wheat many of the same inflammatory properties as sugar. Like sugar, it can also lead to weight gain, belly fat, insulin resistance and chronic digestive disturbances, including irritable bowel syndrome.

What's worse is that a portion of the gluten protein, known as gliadin, has been found to be stimulatory to the brain's receptors, in a similar fashion as opiates. Because of gliadin, eating wheat and wheat-based products can trigger cravings for more and more wheat.

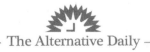

Other gluten-containing grains

As far as other cereal grains, barley and rye are the ones to watch out for most, because they also contain gluten. Even if you don't think you are sensitive to gluten, an inflammatory response in the body is possible. According to Melissa Wood, a nutritional health coach at the the Morrison Center in New York City, "[Gluten] can trigger the immune system, causing inflammation in the intestinal tract."

All in all, if it contains gluten, your best bet is probably to stay away.

Trans fats

Trans fats have long been recognized as the worst type of fats for the body, and, as discussed, have been linked by research to promoting inflammation. These fats are formed when certain oils undergo a process known as hydrogenation, and they are found in many deep-fried foods, baked goods, margarine, lard and shortening.

Along with promoting inflammation, trans fats have been linked to raising LDL "bad" cholesterol and lowering HDL "good" cholesterol, which can cause buildup within artery walls, and contribute to atherosclerosis, the hardening of the arteries. When our arteries are hard and narrow, this spells trouble. Atherosclerosis is a precursor to heart disease, heart attack and stroke.

Additionally, trans fats have been linked to promoting obesity, type 2 diabetes, breast cancer, prostate cancer and Alzheimer's disease.

Processed oils

Highly processed oils, such as canola, vegetable, corn, safflower, sunflower, peanut and soybean oils, may sometimes contain trans fats, which are created as a byproduct

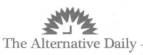

of their processing. Along with the potential for trans fats, these oils contain a large amount of oxidized omega-6 fatty acids.

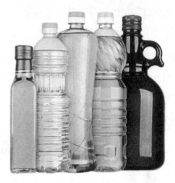

Natural omega-6 fatty acids can be healthy for the body—as long as there are enough omega-3 fatty acids in a specific food to balance them out. When the omega-6 to omega-3 ratio in your body grows too high, inflammation and other health issues may occur.

Too many omega-6 fatty acids, especially in processed form, may raise your risk of high blood pressure, heart disease and autoimmune disorders such as arthritis. Consuming too many of these fatty acids may also promote the growth of certain cancers.

On top of that, highly refined oils do not benefit the body: they are virtually void of nutritional value.

Artificial sweeteners

Artificial sweeteners, used by many people as an alternative to sugar, are not a safe alternative at all. For one thing, many people are sensitive to the chemicals used in these sweeteners, which can cause an inflammatory immune system reaction. Aspartame, a chemical compound synthesized from genetically modified bacteria, is perhaps the most dangerous of these sweeteners.

However, other artificial sweeteners are not safe, either. According to Susie Smithers, a behavioral neuroscientist at Purdue University, individuals who drink soda sweetened

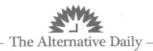

with artificial sweeteners, including aspartame, saccharin and sucralose, are twice as likely to develop metabolic syndrome as people who do not drink this type of soda.

Metabolic syndrome is a term used for a grouping of risk factors, including high blood pressure and abdominal fat, which act as a precursor to heart disease, along with stroke and diabetes. Along with the metabolic syndrome risk, artificial sweeteners can actually lead to the body craving more sugar.

Degraded carrageenan

The inflammatory properties of carrageenan are often overlooked. This is likely because it is made from red seaweed, which in its natural form is incredibly healthy. However, when it is processed and used as a food additive, it can be dangerous.

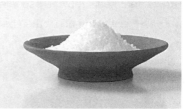

When it is added to foods, processed carrageenan is often not degraded. However, according to some researchers, the acidic environment of the gut may degrade the carrageenan, which can lead to the release of hazardous toxins. Degraded carrageenan itself is actually used to cause inflammation in animal tests.

Watch your food labels closely—many processed and packaged foods, even organics, contain carrageenan.

Processed foods

We've mentioned it before and we'll say it again: any processed food has a high chance of promoting inflammation. Along with the fact that all of the above-listed foods and additives often appear in processed foods—either separately or together—the sheer amount and variety of chemicals, including artificial colors, preservatives, emulsifiers,

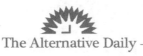

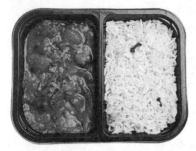

stabilizers and more, deserve no place in your body and may cause an immune system reaction.

To single out two specific examples, artificial colorings have been linked to both inflammation and hormone imbalance. Monosodium glutamate, aka MSG, has also been found to promote chronic inflammation and put a strain on the liver.

Processed meats may be especially dangerous, because along with potentially leading to systemic inflammation, they have also been linked to numerous cancers, including colorectal, pancreatic, stomach, kidney, bladder, lung and testicular cancers, along with leukemia.

Alcohol

While a drink or two per day—one for women, two for men—has actually been linked to health benefits, an excessive amount of alcohol can promote inflammation in multiple organs of the body. It can also weaken liver function, and depending on what you drink, raise blood sugar levels. Plus, there's the nasty addiction factor.

Dairy

While organic dairy products made from the milk of grass-fed animals offer a range of health benefits, conventional versions are often packed with antibiotics, hormones and additives. An excess of dairy may also trigger inflammation due to the presence of casein, which is found in whey protein.

Also, many people are allergic or have a food sensitivity to casein, and this itself may cause an autoimmune reaction.

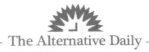

Peanuts

A peanut allergy is one of the most common allergies around today, and if a person with this allergy consumes peanuts, or a processed food that has come into contact with peanuts, a severe inflammatory reaction may occur.

These inappropriately named 'nuts'—since they are actually a legume—can be dangerous for nonallergic individuals as well, because peanuts have a high risk of harboring fungus. If peanuts contaminated with fungus are eaten, inflammation can be triggered.

When it comes to inflammation, avoiding the foods on this list may go far in protecting your health. As far as dairy and peanuts go, they may be alright for some individuals, but be sure to check with a health professional first, and always go for an organic, high-quality variety from a source you trust.

Good food

Just as we don't give unhealthy foods enough credit in contributing to inflammation throughout our bodies, we often don't give healthy foods enough credit for their role in combatting it. All too often, people turn to medications—which can have a number of unwanted side effects—to deal with inflammation and inflammatory pain, and don't give foods the due respect for their healing properties.

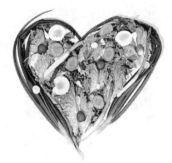

This is a shame, as Mother Nature provides us with an abundance of foods to help stop chronic inflammation at its source. The primary rule is to eat a wide variety of fruits and

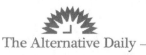

vegetables, along with healthy protein sources, healthy fats and fresh herbs and spices, and to avoid processed foods entirely.

While it would be virtually impossible to list all of the foods that can help fight inflammation, there are a few anti-inflammatory superstars that stand out in the culinary kingdom. The following are the top foods, herbs and spices to add to your diet for maximum inflammation-fighting power.

Hot peppers

Hot peppers, such as chilli peppers and cayenne pepper, contain a wealth of antioxidants, and have been linked by numerous studies to potent anti-inflammatory actions. The active compound in these peppers—which gives them that spicy kick—is known as capsaicin.

When you consume a food high in capsaicin, it triggers an endorphin release in the body, which has been found to help relieve digestive inflammation and the pain of arthritis and neuropathy, to name just two examples.

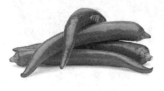

Hot peppers have also been found to help improve circulation, reduce levels of LDL "bad" cholesterol, stabilize blood pressure, and clear blockages from the arteries. All of these factors work together to protect your heart and entire cardiovascular system.

To summarize a 2013 study published in the *International Journal of Immunopathy and Pharmacology*, the authors wrote:

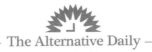

"Several studies have reported that capsaicin is effective in relief and prevention of migraine headaches, improves digestion, helps to prevent heart disease, and lowers blood cholesterol and blood pressure levels. The findings reported in these studies may have implications for the pathophysiology and possible therapy of neuroinflammatory disorders."

Dark green, leafy vegetables

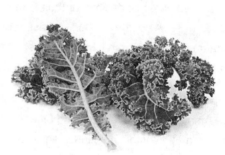

Dark, leafy greens, such as kale, spinach, and collard greens, contain a wide variety of vitamins and minerals, including the famous antioxidant, vitamin C. Vitamin C is well known for protecting the immune system and for combatting inflammation throughout the body. These greens also contain vitamin E, which some research states may protect the body from pro-inflammatory cytokines.

Kale is especially noteworthy for its anti-inflammatory properties, as it has been found to contain over 45 flavonoid antioxidants, including quercetin. These flavonoids work together to keep inflammation at bay. On top of that, kale has significant detoxification abilities, and can even help to flush accumulated inflammatory toxins—such as those which may have built up from eating a Western diet—from the body.

It is noteworthy as well that kale and other cruciferous vegetables contain glucosinolates, compounds which have been linked to aiding in the prevention of a number of cancers.

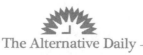

INFLAMMATION ERASED:

NATURALLY FIGHT & REVERSE DAMAGING INFLAMMATORY EFFECTS IN YOUR BODY

Berries

Berries are especially beneficial members of the fruit kingdom because of their super-antioxidant properties. Along with many vitamins and minerals, many berries contain flavonoid antioxidants known as anthocyanins, responsible for their lovely, deep hues. A number of studies have found that anthocyanins can help to combat free radical oxidative stress in the body, thereby reducing inflammation.

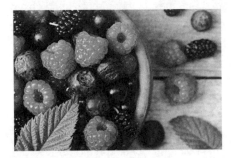

Specifically, strawberries have been linked to lower blood levels of C-reactive protein (a marker of inflammation), and blueberries have been found to protect against the inflammation of the intestines, which characterizes many autoimmune digestive disorders.

Blueberries are actually one of the healthiest berries you can eat—as their concentration of anthocyanins is so high. They also contain resveratrol, an antioxidant compound linked to longevity, and quercetin, another powerful anti-inflammatory antioxidant.

Tart cherries are also of note, due to their high vitamin C content. These berries have been linked to reducing inflammatory muscle pain after exercise, and to reducing the frequency of gout attacks in sufferers of this painful condition.

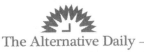

Pineapple

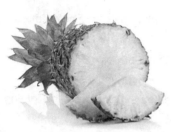

Pineapple, along with other antioxidants, vitamins, and minerals, contains an enzyme called bromelain, which has been found by research to ease inflammatory pain even better than common NSAID medications. It has also been found that this compound can aid in reducing muscle inflammation after a workout.

Due to its high vitamin C content, this is one fruit to stock up on during cold and flu season. In addition to keeping inflammation levels low, it can also help to prevent you from getting sick. If you do get a bug, it may help you to recover faster, as well.

Tomatoes

Tomatoes are noteworthy fighters against inflammation due to their lycopene content. This antioxidant compound has been found to reduce inflammation throughout the body's systems, and specifically in lung tissues. The lycopene in tomatoes is present in both raw and cooked versions.

On lycopene, the authors of a 2013 study published in the *Journal of Nutritional Biochemistry* wrote:

"In moderately overweight, middle-aged subjects, increasing lycopene intake leads to changes to HDL, which we suggest enhanced their antiatherogenic properties. Overall, these results show the heart-protective properties of increased lycopene intake."

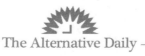

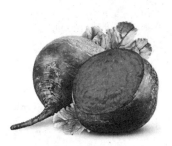

Beets

While most red foods (think berries) are colored red by flavonoid antioxidants such as anthocyanins and carotenoids, beets get their dark color from pigments known as betalains. These pigments contain strong anti-inflammatory properties and are great for fighting free radicals. Beets also contain vitamin C, and a wealth of fiber, among other nutrients.

Wild-caught fatty fish

Fatty fish such as salmon, sardines and mackerel are high in essential omega-3 fatty acids. These fatty acids are called "essential" because they are not produced by the body and must be derived from foods. Omega-3s have been linked to anti-inflammatory, as well as heart and brain protective properties.

Some research has found that people that eat high amounts of foods containing omega-3s have a significantly lower risk of heart disease than people who eat little of these foods.

Flax, chia and hemp seeds

If you are a vegetarian or vegan, or if you just don't like fish, turn to seed sources of omega-3 fatty acids instead. Flax, chia and hemp seeds all contain a wealth of omega-3s in the form of alpha-linolenic acid (ALA). These seeds also contain lignans, which are types of fibers that can help to fight inflammation.

A number of studies have shown that these little seeds can help to protect the cardiovascular system.

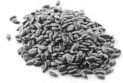

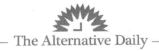

The Alternative Daily

Garlic

Garlic is well known for its antibacterial, antiviral and antifungal properties. These properties are largely attributed to a compound known as allicin, which has also been found to lower the body's production of inflammatory cytokines. Allicin is especially abundant in garlic when it has been chopped or crushed raw, and allowed to sit for several minutes before consuming.

Some research has also found that garlic can help to fight inflammatory pain at a comparable level to NSAID medications.

Onion

Onions are in the same family as garlic, and contain many similar anti-inflammatory properties. They also have a high amount of quercetin and other flavonoid antioxidants. These antioxidants are concentrated in the outer layers of the onion, so don't peel too many of these off when you use them.

Onions also contain allium, which is a potent anti-inflammatory organosulfur compound. Allium not only helps to combat inflammation, but also to reduce the risk of certain cancers and other chronic ailments.

Citrus fruits

Citrus fruits, such as oranges, tangerines, lemons, limes, citrons and grapefruits all contain high levels of vitamin C. Vitamin C is wonderful for keeping your immune system in tip-top shape, and for keeping inflammation down.

Citrus fruits also contain high levels of vitamin A and other carotenoid antioxidants, which have been linked to a lower risk of developing inflammatory-based illnesses.

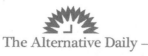

Bee pollen

Bee pollen, made by honeybees themselves, is the synthesis of a male seed of a flower blossom and a bee's digestive enzymes. Many health experts agree that bee pollen is a complete whole food due to its high concentration of protein and ample amount of vitamins (which include B vitamins and vitamin D), minerals and antioxidants.

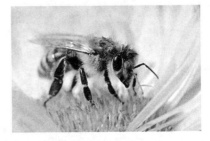

The antioxidants found in bee pollen include both flavonoids and lycopene (also found in tomatoes). On this amazing superfood, the authors of a 2010 study published by BMC wrote:

"It is suggested that the ethanol extract of bee pollen shows a potent anti-inflammatory activity… Some flavonoids included in bee pollen may partly participate in some of the anti-inflammatory action. The bee pollen would be beneficial not only as a dietary supplement but also as a functional food."

Ginger

Ginger, a staple of traditional Ayurvedic medicine, has a unique profile of anti-inflammatory antioxidants. These include gingerols, which have been linked to effectively neutralizing free radicals in the body. It has also been found that ginger is a great alternative to pain medications for inflammatory pain, and can reduce the body's production of pro-inflammatory cytokines.

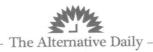

The authors of a 2005 study published in the *Journal of Medicinal Food* wrote:

"The anti-inflammatory properties of ginger have been known and valued for centuries. During the past 25 years, many laboratories have provided scientific support for the long-held belief that ginger contains constituents with anti-inflammatory properties."

Oregano

When it comes to powerhouse antioxidant activity, oregano tops the list. A 2011 study funded by the USDA tested a number of herbs and foods for their antioxidant actions. Oregano—Mexican, Italian and Greek varieties—came out on top. Specifically, oregano was discovered by this study to have 42 times the antioxidant activity of apples, 12 times more than oranges and four times more than blueberries.

A 2012 review published by Cairo University on the properties of oregano reported on several nutritional compounds found in this herb, including carotenoid antioxidants, eight separate flavonoid antioxidants and catechin acid.

Cinnamon

Cinnamon is an ancient spice with potent anti-inflammatory action. The antioxidants in cinnamon are concentrated in its essential oils, including cinnamaldehyde. Other nutrients found in cinnamon bark include B vitamins, vitamins C and E, and a range of minerals.

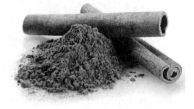

This delicious spice has been linked to increasing insulin sensitivity, lowering blood pressure, and preventing blood platelets from clumping inside arteries. These factors combined make it a wonderful cardioprotective dietary addition indeed.

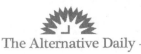

Turmeric

Turmeric is an ancient Indian spice famous for its role in curries. It contains a wealth of anti-inflammatory compounds, including curcumin and curcuminoids. These compounds have been found to manage inflammatory pain in a way that is comparable to NSAID medications. Turmeric has also been linked to turning off a protein in the body that spurs the process of inflammation.

Adding the above-listed foods to a balanced diet of whole, nutritious foods can greatly help you to keep the scourge of inflammation from infiltrating your body. With all of these foods, make sure you choose high-quality, organic varieties whenever possible.

Because foods are highly potent, and not to be underestimated, it is wise to talk to a health professional you trust before consuming any food, herb or spice in large quantities, just to make sure it is safe and recommended for your individual state of health.

Chapter Thirteen
Relieving the Burden of Stress

*I*f you feel stressed, overwhelmed and exhausted just trying to keep up with daily life, and you find yourself flying off the handle or losing control of your emotions regularly, then there is a good chance that a dangerous inflammatory fire is raging in your tissues.

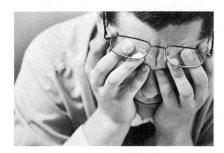

The way you react to life's situations can determine the biochemical triggers that get set

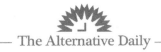

off in your body. Angry, hostile people are shown to have higher levels of C-reactive protein, a molecule which indicates inflammation. Conversely, people who take things in their stride and foster a more relaxed attitude tend not to have as much of this protein in their blood.

The inflammatory response caused by stress can contribute to major chronic illnesses, such as ulcerative colitis. A recent study published in the journal *Gastroenterology Research* reported that extreme stress exposure can multiply the risk of ulcerative colitis episodes up to five times. Most of the leading causes of death in Western countries have now been tied to inflammation, including heart disease, diabetes and cancer.

This can be taken as good news, because it means that all of these killers are largely preventable! However, it is vital to understand the impact of everyday stress and how to take control of it.

Psychological stress causes damage to the body in many ways. A 2013 study shed light on exactly how this happens. Both chronically stressed mice and socioeconomically disadvantaged humans were tested, with similar results. Researchers found that stress changes the genetic activity of immune system cells that are produced in the bone marrow. Before they enter the bloodstream, these cells are prepared to fight infection or trauma, even when there is nothing tangible to fight.

Not only are the cells altered, but more are excreted, too. The study reported that stressed mice had four times the levels of activated immune cells in their blood and spleen compared to non-stressed mice. These "switched on" immune cells exert a pro-inflammatory effect, which affects tissues throughout the body.

An upregulated inflammatory response increases the permeability of the intestines and disrupts neurotransmitters and hormones, contributing to impaired digestion and

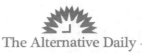

immunity. When your body is functioning in a "high alert" state, it doesn't devote energy to nonessential processes, such as tissue repair and detoxification. Rather, precious resources are spent on building the metabolically expensive stress hormone molecules, such as cortisol and adrenaline.

Although the stress response is intended to function only during acute life-threatening episodes and then to switch off on its own, it often doesn't work that way in modern life. That's why it's vital to purposely and mindfully make an effort to switch off stress and stop the constant firing of stress hormones.

It is undeniable that the mind-body connection is indeed real, and very important for long-term health. Luckily, your stress response is largely under your own control.

It's vital to recognize your own personal stress patterns, and to make conscious changes to improve conditions and relationships which negatively affect you. However, you can also facilitate internal changes, both in the way you respond to stressors and also in how you diffuse the pressure of life's challenges.

There are many ways to manipulate the antistress mechanism in your body. This is called the parasympathetic nervous system. When you are in a calm, relaxed state of mind, bodily resources are put toward digestion, immune system function, tissue repair and reversing inflammation.

The following are some techniques you can use several times a day to unwind, so that inflammation can be healed regularly and does not become a chronic issue manifesting as disease.

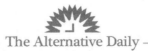

Yoga and other movement

We all know the drill about yoga—it makes you flexible, strong and chilled out. Plus, the fact that yoga and other meditative movement practices have been holding strong in eastern cultures for thousands of years kind of speaks for itself. However, for those who need hard evidence, a 2014 study from the University of Ohio, published in the *Journal of Clinical Oncology*, has uncovered the biochemical underpinnings of these time-honored practices.

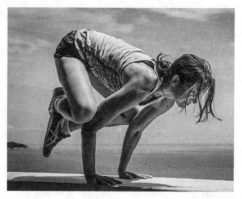

The study participants were 200 breast cancer survivors, half of whom took up yoga for 12 weeks, and half of whom did not. The yoga group reported less fatigue and higher levels of vitality, even three months following the end of the experiment. Blood tests showed that the main three markers of inflammation were reduced by 10 to 15 percent in those who completed the yoga program, as compared to the control group.

A different study, performed on surgical nurses working in stressful situations, found that a yoga program was able to bring about a 40 percent reduction in alpha amylase, a salivary marker of stress.

Some of the mechanisms by which yoga might improve stress response and inflammatory measures are by encouraging deep, rhythmic breathing, stimulating better circulation and digestion, and promoting improved sleep. Yoga can also cross-train your emotional stress response. Another study showed that yogis (term used in reference to those who regularly practice yoga) have less of an inflammatory spike when confronted with a stressful life event, as compared to new practitioners.

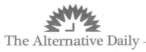

INFLAMMATION ERASED:

NATURALLY FIGHT & REVERSE DAMAGING INFLAMMATORY EFFECTS IN YOUR BODY

Breathing exercises

According to Dr. Andrew Weil, a leading integrative medicine physician, taking a deep breath can positively affect the function of up to 500 genes in one fell swoop. As it happens, breathing is also an important part of yoga, where it is called *pranayama*. This word translates literally as "control of the life force," which indicates that people have been aware of the power of breath to control the body and mind for millennia.

Simple breathing exercises such as "box breathing" can positively influence blood pressure and slow the production of stress hormones. To perform box breathing, simply breathe in for 4 counts, hold for 4, breathe out for 4, hold for 4 and repeat. It's a conscious way that we can tell our brain to put the brakes on stress, and therefore inflammation, too.

Sleep

Not sleeping well puts a major stress load on the body. When we are sleep deprived, we are more irritable and less able to withstand stress or make decisions. There is also a gamut of direct inflammatory effects from inadequate sleep, because this is the time that all sorts of maintenance activities should be happening—things like cell and tissue repair and liver detoxification.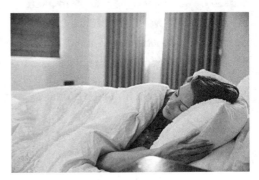

Exercising regularly, getting natural light during the day, and eating foods rich in magnesium are all time-tested strategies for improving the quantity and quality of sleep to support the healing of inflammation.

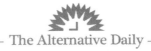

Gratitude

Stress is often a result of dwelling too much on the challenges and inconveniences of daily life. An easy way to overcome this mindset is to practice gratitude. Scientific research supports taking the time to simply write down three things you are thankful for each day. This practice not only relieves stress and curbs inflammation, but also increases happiness to boot.

Time in nature

Many of us spend much of life indoors and trapped in the concrete jungle. Spending time in nature, surrounded by greenery and fresh air, can provide a rapid release from modern-day stresses. Studies show that even looking at an image of an outdoor scene can help reduce stress.

Play and sex

When was the last time you enjoyed a family board game or a game of Frisbee in the park? Finding release through simple, childish play is vital to decompress the pressure of work, bills and the countless other challenges of being an adult.

Intimate time with your partner is another way to disconnect from the stress of the day and stimulate a playful and creative part of the brain. Finally, laughter (not surprisingly) has been demonstrated to be extremely therapeutic, disarming the stress response and soothing inflammation.

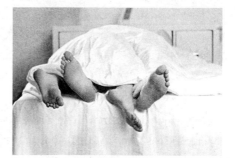

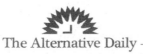

There are so many ways to relieve stress easily and effectively, and most of them can be done entirely free of cost! Try incorporating some of these healthy habits—for their sheer enjoyment, and also with the knowledge that you are preventing the inflammation that causes chronic disease!

Chapter Fourteen
Movement

A s more and more deadly diseases are linked back to inflammation, including Alzheimer's, cancer, diabetes and heart disease, researchers are seeking methods to fight this damaging process. Most of the time, expensive therapies or medications are not needed—we can look to much simpler and more wholesome strategies.

Exercise is one of the holistic ways we can turn down excess inflammation, and scientific research is now supporting this simple intervention.

Studies have found that regular exercise protects against all-cause mortality, mainly by warding off leading causes of death like heart disease and diabetes. As we have covered earlier in this book, these disorders have been associated with chronic low-grade systemic inflammation. Therefore, it seems logical to conclude that exercise protects health by fighting inflammation. Let's dive into the details.

The biochemistry of exercise

Exercise fights inflammation on a molecular level, as demonstrated by a growing body of scientific research. A 2005 study published in the *Journal of Applied Physiology* showed that during exercise, an anti-inflammatory substance called interleukin-6 (IL-6) is produced by contracting muscle fibers. IL-6 stimulates the production of other anti-

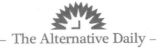

inflammatory compounds called cytokines IL-1ra and IL-10, and at the same time inhibits the production of the proinflammatory cytokine TNF-alpha. In addition, IL-6 enhances the process of burning body fat as energy, by stimulating processes called lipolysis and fat oxidation.

The anti-inflammatory cytokine IL-6, in particular, has been suggested as one of the main protectors against the low-grade inflammation that causes chronic disease. The activity of IL-6 can often be seen by the changes in inflammatory markers after research study participants take part in exercise programs. The main markers that scientists use to measure inflammation are called tumor necrosis factor-alpha (TNF-alpha), C-reactive protein (CRP) and leptin. Leptin is known primarily for its role in appetite suppression, but it can also indicate inflammation, and these two roles are related.

A 2012 study on obese older women (a group very likely to experience chronic inflammation) found that a 12-week resistance training program was able to produce marked improvements in inflammatory markers. Specifically, a 29 percent decrease in TNF-alpha, a 33 percent decrease in CRP and an 18 percent decrease in leptin were observed. There was also a 20 percent increase in IL-10 (interleukin-10), an anti-inflammatory protein.

Finally, the physical strength gained by the study participants (an average of 44 percent over the 12 week period) exhibited benefits, too. The researchers found that there was an inverse relationship between strength and inflammation. The stronger the women were, the lower their inflammatory markers CRP and leptin.

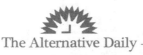

Another way exercise can fight chronic inflammation is by decreasing overall fat mass in the body. As mentioned above, the interleukin-6 produced by muscles during exercise can accelerate the burning of fat as energy. The fat, or adipose tissue, provides a harboring site for toxins and other molecules called adipokines, as well as immune cells called macrophages, which contribute to inflammation. Having less adipose tissue results in a less inflammatory environment overall.

How exercise fights inflammation

Exercise can bring about other positive effects within the body. These can all be tied back to the inflammatory response, conveying direct and indirect benefits.

Improved mood and brain function: Moderate exercise efforts for up to 60 minutes can actually increase positive neurotransmitters, such as serotonin and endorphins, and improve brain chemistry. Moderate intensity exercise also stimulated the growth of new brain cells, neurons and capillary growth to muscles and neurons.

Stress relief: Exercise doesn't have to be strenuous and high impact. Some forms such as swimming, walking and yoga can be restful and meditative. These quieter types of movement can reduce inflammation by relieving mental stress, as well as by improving joint alignment and muscle activation.

Better digestion, elimination and detoxification: Moving your body gets things moving internally, too. This includes food and waste products being worked through your system. Exercise also helps you detoxify accumulated chemical stressors.

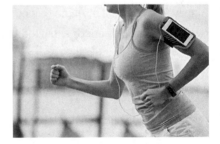

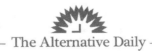

Improved circulation: We all know the exhilarating feeling of getting blood flowing through our veins and air pumping through our lungs. Exercise certainly helps to get blood, oxygen and nutrients circulating throughout tissues and organs to provide for healing processes.

Movement also helps circulate another type of fluid, called lymph. Did you know that your lymph system does not have its own circulatory pump, but rather relies solely on bodily movement, including breathing? It's important to ensure the lymph system does not stagnate, since it plays a key role in shipping out cellular junk and waste products so that they do not stick around and cause illness.

Growth and cell repair: By causing a healthy amount of challenging stress on the body, exercise promotes adaptive regeneration of tissues and the repair of cells so that chronic inflammation does not set in.

Sometimes exercise increases inflammation

Even though physical activity as a whole is considered to be anti-inflammatory, a strenuous workout session actually fires up an acute inflammatory response. Muscles are strained, the cardiovascular system is taxed, and tissues are injured on a microscopic level.

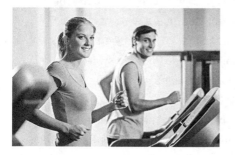

Hold on a second, so exercise can both increase and decrease inflammation? How's that for confusing? Does that mean that challenging exercise is harmful?

As with many things in life, it depends. There are no absolute answers, and the truth falls somewhere in between. Yes, a taxing session

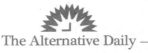

of physical activity incites a sudden, intense bout of inflammation. But this is actually a healthy and necessary step in the process of adaptation that makes the body stronger and more resilient. Without any challenge or stress at all, our muscles and systems would simply languish and waste away. So these short interludes of inflammation from strenuous exercise are beneficial.

In the long run, a robust movement practice is linked with lower levels of inflammation and therefore improved general health.

However, there is one major caveat. Regular exercise can be pro-inflammatory. It becomes that way when the activity is chronic and unrelenting, when for example, a person is training for a marathon and does not take sufficient days to rest and heal between training days. In this case, the acute inflammation that follows a hard workout never has a chance to subside before the next barrage hits.

The takeaway message is that it's highly beneficial to exercise on a regular basis to reduce inflammation, but you must allow time for healing and rebuilding between activity sessions.

A beneficial exercise regimen can take the form of challenging sessions interspersed with days of total rest, or a more regular schedule of less strenuous exercise. This is

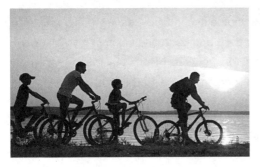

of course very subjective depending on an individual's state of health. For example, a 2013 study on patients with compromised immune systems found that 30 minutes of walking per day, five days per week, was enough exercise to improve inflammatory measures in a safe manner without any detrimental effects.

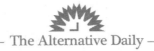

The Alternative Daily

Conversely, for a person in robust health, considerably greater amounts of exercise would likely be safe and beneficial.

Overall, exercise should ideally be varied in type, duration, intensity and frequency. Enjoying a variety of activities on a natural cycle that corresponds with individual needs and energy levels is the best way to reap the considerable anti-inflammatory benefits of exercise.

Physical activity, performed in a conscious and personalized fashion, could contribute to initiatives aimed at reducing chronic inflammatory conditions that plague our society. With the sharing of this knowledge, we hope that this enjoyable, affordable and natural health intervention gains attention and popularity in those hoping to prevent and treat inflammatory diseases. It might even begin to displace some of the more costly, invasive and damaging methods out there today.

Chapter Fifteen
Alternative Therapies and Closing Thoughts

Alternative therapies for inflammation

Western medicine has traditionally viewed inflammation as a dangerous fire that must be put out. We put ice on a sprained ankle to stop the swelling, and block inflammatory receptors with ibuprofen when we have a headache.

As we've covered in this book, many chronic diseases, including our leading causes of death, have now been associated with excess long-term inflammation—so the bad reputation is mostly deserved.

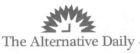

Recently, the picture has become more complex. With more in-depth study, inflammation has been recognized as a vital process for healing. Progressive studies are suggesting that acute inflammation should be allowed to run its course most of the time, because the body has a finely-tuned and highly effective process for immunity, regeneration and healing.

It seems that inflammation is essentially a double-edged sword that must be treated with respect and deliberation. Too little inflammation, and we don't have a properly functioning immune system or cell repair process. Too much, and we end up with a runaway freight train that does endless damage.

However, mainstream medicine still doesn't have the tools to orchestrate the fine balance that is needed in order to keep the inflammatory response correctly tuned. The saying, "when your only tool is a hammer, everything looks like a nail," seems appropriate. Pharmaceutical drugs are like a blunt instrument that just doesn't cut it with the intricate requirements of the human body.

Keeping inflammation in check is really a job for gentler, subtler, holistic therapies. Along with a conscious, responsible, preventative lifestyle, of course.

The following are some of the most promising natural and traditional modalities that can be used to treat excess inflammation.

Herbal medicine

Plants such as herbs and spices contain an amazing number of medicinal compounds. A 2010 study performed in Vienna, Austria, published in the journal *Food Chemistry*, tested several plants for anti-inflammatory abilities and found that the inflammatory proteins interleukin-6 (IL-6) and tumor necrosis factor-alpha (TNF-A) were dramatically reduced, while anti-inflammatory interleukin-10 was increased.

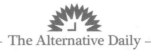

According to the Austrian study, the highest anti-inflammatory potential was found in chilli pepper, with its active constituent capsaicin. Other plants that were able to improve inflammatory profiles were allspice, basil, bay leaves, black pepper, licorice, nutmeg, oregano, sage and thyme. Similarly, turmeric is highly celebrated as a therapeutic spice.

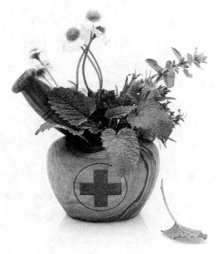

Another recent study examined the function of plant compounds called flavonoids as antioxidant and antiproliferative medicines against inflammation and major diseases. Flavonoids are found in high quantities in seeds, citrus fruits, olive oil, tea and red wine. The researchers pointed out that flavonoids found in plants have a high efficacy rate and excellent safety record, having been used in Eastern medicine for thousands of years. However, these compounds have yet to find a significant place within Western medicine.

A further study from the University of South Carolina Cancer Center used advanced molecular biology to analyze and support the ability of various phytochemicals (plant compounds) to treat or manage "a plethora of modern diseases," including many different cancers and chronic inflammatory illnesses.

Overall, incorporating a wide variety of fruits, vegetables, herbs, spices, nuts, seeds, unprocessed plant oils and teas into your diet will ensure that you have a consistent intake of all the powerful therapeutic compounds offered by the rich world of plants.

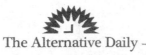

Aromatherapy

While essential oils have been used in traditional medicine for ages, scientific research on their activity and efficacy has only taken place in the last few decades. Essential oils are potent extracts of the roots, bark, seeds, leaves or resins of plants, derived via steam distillation or pressing.

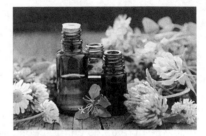

While the scents of essential oils have a profound effect on the brain and stress response, the oils can also be used topically on the skin, where they may exert analgesic (pain-relieving), antispasmodic, anti-inflammatory and antirheumatic properties.

Essential oils can be used in a number of different ways. You can simply breathe in their scents, mix them into a bath, use them for massage or apply them to a comforting hot or cold compress. These gentle methods may make excellent alternatives to anti-inflammatory treatments such as cortisone, which can have concerning side effects.

Some essential oils that are traditionally used for calming inflammation include chamomile, lavender, copaiba, palo santo, eucalyptus, peppermint, clary sage and frankincense. A 2005 study examined the efficacy of 77 different essential oils, highlighting oregano, lemongrass and melaleuca (tea tree) as good choices for treating excessive inflammation.

It is thought that essential oils act intelligently in the body, destroying ailing cells but leaving healthy ones untouched.

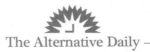

It is important to note that essential oils are very potent, and some require distillation before direct application to the skin. It is best to consult a natural health professional before using essential oils at home—and always purchase high-quality, therapeutic grade oils from a source you trust.

Acupuncture

The therapeutic value of acupuncture has been undoubted by millions of beneficiaries and practitioners for thousands of years, and this is now being confirmed by scientific studies.

A 2014 study published in *Nature Medicine* examined the treatment of hospital patients with an inflammatory condition called sepsis, which causes 250,000 deaths each year in the United States. The researchers used acupuncture to stimulate the vagus nerve,

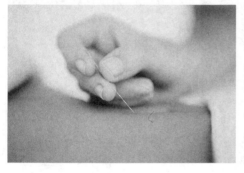

which is the major pathway connecting the brainstem to the gut. It was observed that this vagal stimulation was able to activate bodily mechanisms which reduce inflammation.

This type of treatment holds promise for other inflammatory diseases as well, including arthritis and Crohn's disease.

Massage therapy

It's undeniable that a good massage relieves stress, which can dampen inflammatory mechanisms in the body. This is supported by a 2012 study from McMaster University, where it was found that tissues receiving massage produced lower amounts of inflammatory proteins.

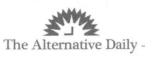

These changes were caused by altered gene activity in relation to inflammation, both immediately after massage and later in the recovery process. The researchers also found that massage was associated with increased expression of PGC-1-alpha, which is a molecule that helps with tissue repair.

This important evidence supports the use of massage both as a preventative therapy and also to aid in the healing of more acute conditions.

Eastern medicine

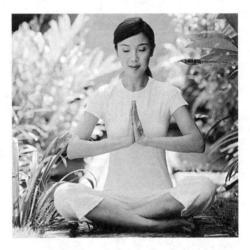

Some of the most prominent traditions in Eastern medicine include Ayurveda and Traditional Chinese Medicine (TCM). These medical systems operate on principles of energy, balance and flow within the body. Meditation is an important practice in Eastern medicine. Robust scientific evidence supports its ability to calm the stress response, and as a result, control unhealthy inflammation.

Eastern medical modalities make frequent use of adaptogenic herbs, which are considered a panacea for stress and inflammation. Ayurveda favors ashwagandha and holy basil, while TCM recommends ginseng root, schizandra berry or reishi mushroom. These herbs are thought to have an intelligent nonspecific effect in the body, meaning they will provide just what an individual needs at a particular time in order to find balance.

Ayurvedic and Chinese medical practices highlight the importance of eating the appropriate foods for an individual's condition, while encouraging detoxification and

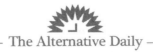

gentle movement. This holistic approach is light years ahead of its time, and provides an excellent model to follow in terms of taking control of inflammation to prevent disease.

Note: As many of the remedies recommended in traditional medicines can be highly potent, it is best to use them under the guidance of a knowledgeable natural health professional.

Homeopathy

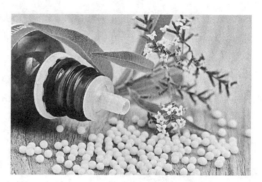

This type of therapy is based on the concept of "like dissolves like." Small doses of remedies which resemble diseases are used to stimulate healing. Arnica is commonly used to curb inflammation, as are bryonia, belladonna and apis. The specialized action eopathic treatments can be used for addressing specific ailments, while a complementary regime of anti-inflammatory food, rest and gentle exercise should be undertaken to facilitate healing.

Working with a skilled practitioner is the best way to experience the benefits of homeopathic treatment.

Why not experiment with the wide range of natural and holistic remedies available to you before resorting to the harsh and invasive mechanisms of pharmaceutical drugs? If you find a couple of alternative therapies that work for you, try incorporating them into a regular preventative routine, so that you can keep inflammation in check thereby keeping your body strong and healthy.

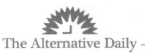

Closing Thought: Your Health is In Your Hands!

While we cannot predict the future, and disease may sometimes strike despite our best efforts, the quality of our health is largely up to us. Chronic inflammation is a very real and prevalent danger—one which many ignore until disease strikes. To keep your body and mind as healthy and happy as possible, the time to adopt a healthy, holistic lifestyle is now.

Choosing to to begin living a healthy life today is one of the best decisions you can make for yourself, and for those you care for. By taking steps to keep your inflammation levels in check, you may even be able to prevent a host of diseases from setting in and taking their toll. We only get one body: if you provide it the nourishment, movement and gentle care that it needs, it will likely serve you kindly for years to come.

We wish you the best of luck on your journey!

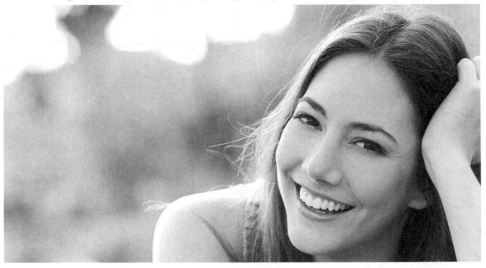

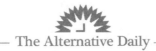

Sources

1. http://www.cdc.gov/heartdisease/facts.htm

2. http://myheartsisters.org/2010/07/17/heart-disease-countries/

3. http://www.healthline.com/health/heart-disease/statistics

4. http://www.npr.org/sections/thesalt/2014/03/28/295332576/why-we-got-fatter-during-the-fat-free-food-boom

5. http://millionhearts.hhs.gov/abouthds/cost-consequences.html

6. http://www.thennt.com/nnt/statins-for-heart-disease-prevention-without-prior-heart-disease/

7. http://www.ncbi.nlm.nih.gov/pubmed/21249663

8. http://www.webmd.com/heart-disease/common-medicine-heart-disease-patients?page=2

9. http://my.chriskresser.com/wp-content/uploads/membership-files/ebooks/Diet%20Heart%20Myth.pdf

10. http://www.ncbi.nlm.nih.gov/pubmed/22231607

11. http://archinte.jamanetwork.com/article.aspx?articleid=1108676&resultclick=3

12. http://www.fda.gov/downloads/ForConsumers/ConsumerUpdates/UCM293705.pdf

13. http://www.ncbi.nlm.nih.gov/pubmed/20488911

14. http://www.cmaj.ca/content/181/1-2/E11.abstract

15. http://www.ncbi.nlm.nih.gov/pmc/articles/PMC4113766/

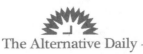

16. http://www.ncbi.nlm.nih.gov/pubmed/21475195

17. http://content.onlinejacc.org/article.aspx?articleid=1920817&resultClick=3

18. http://www.ncbi.nlm.nih.gov/pubmed/21807932

19. http://www.ncbi.nlm.nih.gov/pmc/articles/PMC3322682/

20. http://content.onlinejacc.org/article.aspx?articleid=1856901

21. http://www.medicalnewstoday.com/articles/290747.php

22. http://www.biomedcentral.com/1471-2431/7/36/

23. http://molpharm.aspetjournals.org/content/73/2/399.short

24. http://www.sciencedirect.com/science/article/pii/S0308814610003158

25. http://www.worldscientific.com/doi/abs/10.1142/S0192415X09006734

26. http://www.jivaresearch.org/research/curcumin/From_ancient_medicine_to_modern_
     medicine-_Ayurvedic_concepts_of_health_and_their_role_in_inflamma.pdf

27. http://pharmrev.aspetjournals.org/content/52/4/673.short

28. http://www.sciencedirect.com/science/article/pii/S0889157506000196

29. http://link.springer.com/article/10.1007/BF00916043

30. http://onlinelibrary.wiley.com/doi/10.1002/biof.5520130123/abstract

31. http://www.sciencedirect.com/science/article/pii/S0962456204000906

32. http://www.sciencedirect.com/science/article/pii/S0962456201800394

33. http://opensiuc.lib.siu.edu/ebl/vol2008/iss1/78/

34. http://www.hindawi.com/journals/mi/2003/807126/abs/

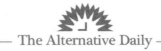

35. http://www.ncbi.nlm.nih.gov/pmc/articles/PMC3632662/

36. http://stm.sciencemag.org/content/4/119/119ra13.short

37. http://www.ncbi.nlm.nih.gov/pubmed/15772055

38. http://content.onlinejacc.org/article.aspx?articleid=1132588

39. http://www.ncbi.nlm.nih.gov/pubmed/17144883

40. http://www.nature.com/nri/journal/v11/n9/full/nri3041.html

41. http://www.nature.com/nrrheum/journal/v11/n2/full/nrrheum.2014.193.html

42. http://jasn.asnjournals.org/content/early/2014/04/02/ASN.2013070702

43. http://jap.physiology.org/content/103/1/376

44. http://journals.lww.com/epidem/Abstract/2002/09000/Does_Exercise_Reduce_Inflammation__Physical.12.aspx

45. http://www.hindawi.com/journals/mi/2010/171023/

46. http://www.ncbi.nlm.nih.gov/pubmed/12192226

47. http://www.ncbi.nlm.nih.gov/pubmed/19695853

48. http://www.ncbi.nlm.nih.gov/pubmed/21970447

49. http://journals.lww.com/acsm-msse/Abstract/2009/08000/A_Yearlong_Exercise_Intervention_Decreases_CRP.1.aspx

50. http://www.ncbi.nlm.nih.gov/pmc/articles/PMC1087185/

51. https://www.era-edta.org/ekha/WHO_Global_Status_Report_on_NCDs_2014.pdf

52. http://www.diabetes.org/diabetes-basics/statistics/

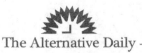

53. http://www.cdc.gov/diabetes/data/statistics/2014statisticsreport.html

54. http://www.cdc.gov/nchs/fastats/deaths.htm

55. http://diabetes.diabetesjournals.org/content/52/3/812.long

56. http://jama.jamanetwork.com/article.aspx?articleid=1832542

57. http://www.cdc.gov/features/diabetesfactsheet/

58. http://www.ama-assn.org/sub/prevent-diabetes-stat/index.html?utm_
    source=(direct)&utm_medium=(none)&utm_term=vanity&utm_content=prediabetes_
    stat&utm_campaign=partnership

59. http://www.ncbi.nlm.nih.gov/pubmed/16613757

60. http://www.diabetes.org/diabetes-basics/type-1/?loc=db-slabnav

61. http://jdrf.org/about-jdrf/fact-sheets/type-1-diabetes-facts/

62. http://www.ncbi.nlm.nih.gov/pmc/articles/PMC1892523/

63. http://www.sciencedirect.com/science/article/pii/S0168822714001879

64. http://www.cdc.gov/pcd/issues/2014/13_0415.htm

65. http://journals.cambridge.org/action/displayAbstract?fromPage=online&aid=9888262&file
    Id=S0007114515002093

66. http://www.ncbi.nlm.nih.gov/pmc/articles/PMC3827123/

67. http://www.jleukbio.org/content/95/1/149.abstract

68. http://www.niddk.nih.gov/health-information/health-topics/diagnostic-tests/a1c-test-
    diabetes/Pages/index.aspx

69. http://www.cdc.gov/diabetes/basics/diabetes.html

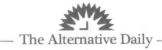

70. http://www.ncbi.nlm.nih.gov/pmc/articles/PMC4287776/

71. http://www.bmj.com/content/343/bmj.d4169.full

72. http://www.ncbi.nlm.nih.gov/pubmed?term=%22The+New+England+journal+of+medicine%22%5bJour%5d+AND+2007/05/21%5bpdat%5d+AND+Nissen%5bauthor

73. http://www.drugwatch.com/actos/treating-type-2-diabetes-with-medication/

74. http://www.diabetes.org/food-and-fitness/?loc=ff-slabnav

75. http://www.nature.com/nature/journal/v392/n6674/full/392398a0.html

76. http://www.ncbi.nlm.nih.gov/pmc/articles/PMC2829991/

77. http://www.niddk.nih.gov/about-niddk/research-areas/diabetes/diabetes-prevention-program-dpp/Pages/default.aspx

78. http://www.cdc.gov/diabetes/living/eatright.html

79. http://www.niddk.nih.gov/health-information/health-topics/weight-control/just-enough/Pages/just-enough-for-you.aspx

80. http://jn.nutrition.org/content/132/9/2488.short

81. http://www.mayoclinic.org/healthy-lifestyle/nutrition-and-healthy-eating/in-depth/high-fiber-foods/art-20050948

82. http://www.ncbi.nlm.nih.gov/pubmed/24512603

83. http://www.cdc.gov/HealthyYouth/publications/pdf/PP-Ch7.pdf

84. http://www.cdc.gov/diabetes/living/beactive.html

85. http://www.niddk.nih.gov/news/research-updates/Pages/health-effects-diet-exercise-adults-type-2-diabetes-obesity.aspx

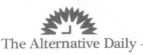

86. http://mcr.aacrjournals.org/content/4/4/221.full.html

87. http://www.biooncology.com/molecular-causes-of-cancer/inflammation

88. http://www.ncbi.nlm.nih.gov/pmc/articles/PMC1994795/

89. http://www.nature.com/nature/journal/v420/n6917/full/nature01322.html

90. http://link.springer.com/chapter/10.1007/0-387-26283-0_1

91. http://www.ncbi.nlm.nih.gov/pmc/articles/PMC3332223/

92. http://carcin.oxfordjournals.org/content/30/7/1073.full

93. http://news.emory.edu/stories/2014/03/chemo_inflammation_epigenetics_breast_cancer_survivors/index.html

94. http://www.cell.com/abstract/S0092-8674(10)00060-7

95. http://www.sciencedirect.com/science/article/pii/S0140673600040460

96. http://www.researchgate.net/publication/6896641_Inflammation_and_cancer_How_hot_is_the_link

97. http://www.bloodjournal.org/content/126/5/582?sso-checked=true

98. http://www.springer.com/us/book/9781461468189

99. http://www.ncbi.nlm.nih.gov/pubmed/15766659/

100. http://www.ncbi.nlm.nih.gov/pubmed/11229684/

101. http://www.ncbi.nlm.nih.gov/pubmed/18987874/

102. http://www.ncbi.nlm.nih.gov/pubmed/16967326/

103. http://www.medicalnewstoday.com/articles/247459.php

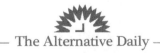

104. http://www.eurekalert.org/pub_releases/2015-04/uops-cc041615.php

105. http://www.scientificamerican.com/article/chronic-inflammation-cancer/

106. http://www.hopkinsmedicine.org/news/media/releases/chronic_inflammation_linked_to_high_grade_prostate_cancer

107. http://www.sciencedaily.com/releases/2011/04/110419091159.htm

108. http://www.journal-inflammation.com/content/11/1/23

109. http://www.cell-symposia-cancerandinflammation.com/

110. http://www.medicalnewstoday.com/articles/248423.php

111. http://scienceblog.cancerresearchuk.org/2013/02/01/feeling-the-heat-the-link-between-inflammation-and-cancer/

112. http://newsoffice.mit.edu/2015/link-between-inflammation-and-cancer-0115

113. http://www.nature.com/nature/journal/v420/n6917/full/nature01322.html

114. http://www.cancernetwork.com/review-article/chronic-inflammation-and-cancer

115. http://www.mdanderson.org/patient-and-cancer-information/cancer-information/cancer-topics/prevention-and-screening/food/inflammationandcancer.html

116. http://www.ncbi.nlm.nih.gov/pmc/articles/PMC3538397/

117. http://www.dailymail.co.uk/health/article-1184289/Can-cancer-drugs-harm-memory-Patients-complain-mental-problems-chemo.html

118. http://www.sciencedirect.com/science/article/pii/S0889159114000567

119. http://www.mayoclinic.org/diseases-conditions/cancer/basics/risk-factors/con-20032378

120. http://www.ncbi.nlm.nih.gov/pubmed/21219177

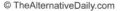
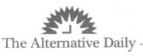

121. http://www.ncsf.org/enew/articles/articles-obesityandinflammation.aspx

122. https://chriskresser.com/how-inflammation-makes-you-fat-and-diabetic-and-vice-versa/

123. http://www.jci.org/articles/view/57132

124. http://www.ncbi.nlm.nih.gov/pubmed/21481713

125. http://www.journal-inflammation.com/content/7/1/35

126. http://www.hindawi.com/journals/isrn/2013/697521/

127. http://www.thelancet.com/journals/lancet/article/PIIS0140-6736(14)60460-8/abstract

128. http://www.webmd.com/diet/20140528/obesity-overweight-rates-jump-worldwide-report-finds?src=RSS_PUBLIC

129. http://diabetes.diabetesjournals.org/content/57/6/1470.full

130. http://www.webmd.com/diet/20121212/whey-amino-acids-fat-loss

131. http://www.aminoacid-studies.com/areas-of-use/fat-burning.html

132. http://www.heart.org/HEARTORG/GettingHealthy/NutritionCenter/HealthyDietGoals/Sugars-and-Carbohydrates_UCM_303296_Article.jsp

133. http://ajcn.nutrition.org/content/94/2/479.short

134. http://www.plantphysiol.org/content/66/5/950.full.pdf

135. http://www.mdpi.com/2072-6643/5/3/771/htm

136. http://www.ncbi.nlm.nih.gov/pubmed/12580703

137. http://onlinelibrary.wiley.com/doi/10.1111/j.1745-4522.1994.tb00244.x/abstract

138. http://www.medicalnewstoday.com/articles/237191.php

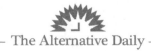

139. https://www.nhlbi.nih.gov/health/health-topics/topics/heartattack

140. http://www.sott.net/article/242516-Heart-surgeon-speaks-out-on-what-really-causes-heart-disease

141. http://www.arthritis.org/about-arthritis/types/

142. http://rheumatology.oxfordjournals.org/content/38/11/1039.full

143. http://www.niams.nih.gov/health_info/rheumatic_disease/

144. http://www.rheumatology.org/I-Am-A/Patient-Caregiver/Diseases-Conditions/Rheumatoid-Arthritis

145. http://www.arthritis.org/about-arthritis/understanding-arthritis/

146. http://www.ncbi.nlm.nih.gov/pubmed/24192039

147. http://www.arthritis.org/living-with-arthritis/arthritis-diet/foods-to-avoid-limit/food-ingredients-and-inflammation.php

148. http://www.medicalnewstoday.com/articles/7621.php

149. http://www.ncbi.nlm.nih.gov/pubmed/12442909

150. http://nationalmirroronline.net/new/sedentary-lifestyle-major-cause-of-arthritis-physiotherapist/

151. http://www.arthritis.org/living-with-arthritis/comorbidities/depression-and-arthritis/stress-rheumatoid-arthritis.php

152. http://www.ncbi.nlm.nih.gov/pubmed/21893478

153. http://www.ncbi.nlm.nih.gov/pmc/articles/PMC3257638/

154. http://www.ncbi.nlm.nih.gov/pmc/articles/PMC2291500/

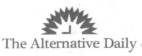

155. http://www.healthdata.org/news-release/deaths-cardiovascular-disease-increase-globally-while-mortality-rates-decrease

156. http://www.who.int/mediacentre/factsheets/fs310/en/

157. http://press.endocrine.org/doi/10.1210/jc.2015-1677

158. http://www.who.int/mediacentre/news/releases/2003/pr27/en/

159. http://care.diabetesjournals.org/content/24/11/1936.long

160. http://www.cdc.gov/nchs/data/databriefs/db10.pdf

161. http://www.who.int/mediacentre/news/releases/2012/dementia_20120411/en/

162. http://www.pcrm.org/media/online/sept2014/seven-foods-to-supercharge-your-gut-bacteria

163. https://chriskresser.com/is-gerd-an-autoimmune-disease/

164. http://www.cdc.gov/fungal/diseases/candidiasis/

165. http://www.theibsnetwork.org/what-is-ibs/

166. https://www.crohnsandcolitis.com/crohns/what-is-crohns-disease

167. https://www.crohnsandcolitis.com/crohns/inside-inflammation

168. http://www.ccfa.org/what-are-crohns-and-colitis/what-is-crohns-diseasehttp://www.ccfa.org/what-are-crohns-and-colitis/what-is-crohns-disease/types-of-crohns-disease.html?referrer=http://www.ccfa.org/what-are-crohns-and-colitis/what-is-crohns-disease/

169. https://www.crohnsandcolitis.com/crohns/disease-diagnosis

170. https://celiac.org/celiac-disease/what-is-celiac-disease/

171. https://celiac.org/celiac-disease/symptomssigns/

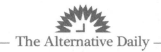

172. http://www.health.harvard.edu/staying-healthy/foods-that-fight-inflammation

173. http://www.med.monash.edu.au/cecs/gastro/prebiotic/faq/#6

174. http://www.drperlmutter.com/eat/brain-maker-foods/

175. http://www.hindawi.com/journals/grp/2013/653989/

176. http://www.ncbi.nlm.nih.gov/pmc/articles/PMC2879816/

177. http://www.ncbi.nlm.nih.gov/pmc/articles/PMC3667473/

178. http://www.healthline.com/health/gerd/genetics

179. http://www.sts.org/patient-information/esophageal-surgery/gastroesophageal-reflux-disease

180. http://www.nlm.nih.gov/medlineplus/gerd.html

181. http://www.mayoclinic.org/diseases-conditions/gerd/basics/symptoms/con-20025201

182. http://www.mayoclinic.org/diseases-conditions/gerd/basics/lifestyle-home-remedies/con-20025201

183. http://www.mayoclinic.org/diseases-conditions/gerd/basics/treatment/con-20025201

184. http://www.mayoclinic.org/diseases-conditions/gerd/basics/alternative-medicine/con-20025201

185. http://www.thedailybeast.com/articles/2015/04/28/the-cure-for-brain-diseases-is-in-your-gut.html

186. http://www.thecandidadiet.com/inflammation-candida-gut-flora/

187. http://www.thecandidadiet.com/what-is-candida-albicans/

188. http://www.webmd.com/oral-health/tc/thrush-cause

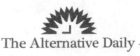

189. http://www.mayoclinic.org/diseases-conditions/yeast-infection/basics/prevention/con-20035129

190. http://www.cdc.gov/cfs/symptoms/index.html

191. http://hivinsite.ucsf.edu/InSite%3Fpage%3Dkb-00%26doc%3Dkb-05-02-03

192. http://www.ncbi.nlm.nih.gov/pubmed/15907554

193. http://www.ncbi.nlm.nih.gov/pubmed/12839324

194. http://www.webmd.com/skin-problems-and-treatments/candidiasis

195. http://www.ncbi.nlm.nih.gov/pubmed/17651080

196. https://www.kingbio.com/aquaflora/candida-test

197. http://www.ncbi.nlm.nih.gov/pmc/articles/PMC3667473/

198. http://www.diabetes.org/are-you-at-risk/diabetes-risk-test/

199. http://www.cdc.gov/diabetes/prevention/pdf/prediabetestest.pdf

200. http://patient.info/health/blood-tests-to-detect-inflammation

201. http://www.ewg.org

202. http://www.grassrootshealth.net/garland02-11

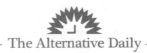

The Alternative Daily